# THE KETAMINE HANDBOOK

# CONTENTS

# PROLOGUE

Once upon a time, there was a girl who had a very, very bad case of depression. She made many attempts to get help. She tried a number of different drugs, all of which made her feel profoundly worse. She tried a number of different therapies, to no avail. She even tried hospitalization, only to quickly realize that in doing so, she found herself in a terrifying system that stripped away all of her rights and comforts.

She looked for any kind of support—for any kind of resource that could help her—and found little to none. She tried talking to her family and friends but no one seemed to understand.

*Why had nothing worked?* she wondered. *What is wrong with me? Can I ever get better? Is this how it's always going to be?*

Sound familiar? Chances are there are probably quite a few of you who can relate to this: a 2021 study found that 2.8 million Americans had treatment-resistant depression (Zhdanava et al. 2021). And this little excerpt of a story is only the tip of the iceberg. Many adults with treatment-resistant depression will turn to a number of poor behaviors in an attempt to cope with their condition. This could include anything from substance abuse to self-harm and even suicide.

I wanted to write this book because I am that girl. I've suffered from treatment-resistant depression for a long, long time and found no relief no matter what I did. I had reached a point of desperation and futility where I felt everything was over; that no matter what I did, I could not, for some reason, "unfuck" my brain.

I'm here to write this book today, however, thanks to a number of health-care providers that saved my life. But before I could get the care I needed, I had to step into a place of fear.

The first time I was exposed to ketamine was at a house party in the UK in 2012. Everyone was going around huffing fat lines of ket, and they all seemed so jolly at first...

And then I saw one of the guys on the floor using his arms to crawl across the carpet, screaming, "GUYS, WHERE ARE MY LEGS? I THINK I LEFT THEM BEHIND, CAN YOU HELP ME FIND THEM?"

I was horrified, and vowed right then and there to never touch ketamine.

So when my health-care provider suggested ketamine might be a viable option for my treatment-resistant depression a couple of years ago, you can imagine the fear I felt. I didn't know what to expect, or how the drug would affect me. I had only ever known about it through word of mouth stories or at parties where it was abused. Stories of "K-holes," or states where users would take so much ketamine they'd be totally unresponsive, spread like wildfire. My preconceived notions about the drug—the stigma it carried— nearly prevented me from even giving it a try.

I did, however, manage to overcome that fear, and I'm so, so glad I did, because without it, I might not be here today.

I wanted to share this story with you in the hopes that it might inspire some of you to finally go out and take that first step. I know how scary it can be, and I know how scared of ketamine I used to be. But if the cure to depression lies in neuroplasticity—in our ability to

create new pathways for ourselves, new ways to approach things—
then the only way to improve is to step into the unknown.

I hope you don't let fear run your life like I did. I hope that you don't
let stigmas stop you from getting the care you deserve. I hope you
find the right way forward.

For those of you who feel ketamine may be a viable treatment
option for you, I've included as much detail as I can detailing how
you can get access to ketamine treatment/therapy. The information
in chapter 5, Accessing Ketamine Therapy (see page 96), is derived
from my years of trying to get ketamine treatment covered by an
insurance provider as well as from anecdotal reports from social
media sites like Reddit. I've included tips for navigating insurance
providers, tips from psychiatrists on finding the right provider,
and a comprehensive database listing all the ketamine treatment
providers I could find. Please note, however, that I am merely one
human being, and this information may be limited in certain places.
I have done my best because I believe you deserve it.

# INTRODUCTION

## WHAT IS KETAMINE?

Sometimes referred to as "Special K" or simply as a horse tranquilizer, ketamine is often thought of as a rave or clubbing drug. Many of us are all too familiar with this negative modern-day assumption about ketamine. While ketamine is used recreationally, this application of the compound deviates significantly from its original intended use.

So what was ketamine's original use, anyway? How did this drug first come to be, and how did it earn this reputation? Is ketamine friend or foe?

This book is designed to answer all of those questions, and then some.

We'll begin by dispelling popular negative stereotypes and assumptions about ketamine with a little history lesson in chapter 1. How did these negative stereotypes about ketamine first enter popular culture? We'll discuss how this compound came into existence and learn more about its initial medical uses. As we continue to investigate, we'll dive into an analysis of how the popular misconceptions/beliefs about ketamine originated and spread across the country in tandem with public perception and policy.

Once you have an idea of how ketamine came to earn its bad rap, we'll dive into the science of this unique compound in chapter 2,

"What Is Ketamine & How Does It Work?" In chapters 3 and 4, we'll discuss ketamine's promising clinical applications, including ketamine-assisted psychotherapy (KAP), before I include some practical tips on how to access ketamine treatment for yourself in chapter 5. And finally, we'll round out the whole discussion with chapter 6, on the future of ketamine, in which we discuss patents, new methodologies, and exciting clinical applications on the horizon. What does the future hold in store for us?

I spent the last year condensing hundreds of research papers, journal articles, interviews, firsthand reports, fact sheets, case reports, and more into one book written in simple, easy-to-understand language. It's my gift to you.

Now go forth and unfuck thyself.

# Chapter 1

# SAY HELLO TO THE NEW DRUG ON THE BLOCK: KETAMINE

Welcome to this great-big little book all about drugs—specifically, ketamine.

Before we get into all of the good stuff, I'd like you to humor me for a moment.

What do you think of when you hear the term "PCP"?

I'll wait.

Did your answer contain some version of "superhuman strength"? How about the word "rampage"? Whatever the phrases that popped into your head, chances are they weren't particularly pro-PCP.

Commonly known as angel dust, phencyclidine, or PCP, has earned a legendary reputation for its pronounced, bizarre effects. These can include feelings of invincibility and mind-bending mania, hallmarks of stories about PCP trips gone horribly wrong.

You might be thinking, *Wow, how did such a nefarious drug ever end up in public hands?* Or perhaps you're busy pondering what PCP has to do with ketamine. More on that soon.

PCP, funnily enough, started out as a drug with clear medical usage as an anesthetic. Anesthetic drugs are utilized during surgeries to induce a loss of sensation. This includes a loss of consciousness as well as antinociceptive effects (loss of pain).

PCP was first synthesized in 1956 by chemists at the Parke-Davis company. While it functioned as a safe and reliable anesthetic agent, PCP also came with a litany of, well, less-than-desirable effects—most notably, delirium. Delirium refers to extreme, serious disturbances in mental abilities and cognition. In PCP's case, this delirium manifested as "degrees of manic behavior" and "halluci-nations with distortion of vision" (Domino et al. 1965). Researchers also noted PCP reactions seemed to depend on several factors, including gender. While women tended to experience a happy drunken state (Greifenstein 1958), men under its effects were found to be "violent and aggressive to a degree which requires constant supervision for up to three hours" (Johnstone et al. 1959).

Desperate for answers, scientists began searching for a suitable PCP substitute, one that would anesthetize patients without the troubling side effects. Their answer wouldn't arrive until 1962, which was the year that Calvin Stevens, an organic chemist and Parke-Davis consultant, developed what we now know as ketamine (Domino 1980).

Initially identified as CI-581, ketamine is a structural analog of PCP. This means the two compounds have similar structures with a few notable differences. Despite the similarity in structure, ketamine was found to be far less potent than PCP—specifically, one-tenth the potency—and so ketamine was subsequently selected for human trials moving forward (Li and Vlisides 2016).

The first human anesthetic dose of ketamine was administered in 1964 by two University of Michigan professors, Dr. Edward Domino of pharmacology and Dr. Guenter Corssen of anesthesiology. The two administered ketamine to 20 humans and concluded the drug was a viable, safe, and effective option for clinical anesthetic use (Domino 1980).

Domino and Corssen published the first clinical study of ketamine as a human anesthetic in 1966, reporting its anesthetic effects in 130 patients aged 6 weeks to 86 years across 133 surgical procedures (Corssen and Domino 1966). What they discovered would go on to shape the future of anesthetic medicine as we know it today.

# DISSOCIATIVE ANESTHESIA

Ketamine was found to produce novel states in which patients might *appear* to be awake but were unable to respond to sensory input. Domino's wife called this state "dissociative anesthesia." Ketamine produced highly altered states of consciousness coupled with "profound analgesia," or painkilling effects in patients. Anesthesiology is a medical specialty that centers around the care of patients before, during, and after surgery. Being able to induce anesthesia, a state in which patients lose awareness of their surroundings, is one vital component of anesthesiology. Unlike PCP, however, it had minimal side effects, most notably a lack of severe delirium (Corssen and Domino 1966).

Dissociation isn't as uncommon as you might think. In fact, chances are you've probably experienced some form of dissociation before; it's a common type of defense mechanism in which your brain seems to disconnect you from the world around you. This can create the strange sensation that you are an observer, watching life around you unfurl without taking a part in all the action. In this state, time can even appear to stand still. The addition of an analgesic component can produce additional feelings of euphoria as the body becomes free of residual aches and pains.

Domino and Corssen's report would go on to make ketamine one of the most popular induction agents among anesthesiologists. Ketamine wasn't just for adult humans, either. It was also adopted into veterinary and pediatric anesthesia practices as it proved to be a useful sedating agent for less-than-cooperative patients such as children and animals.

Ketamine, funnily enough, wasn't the only mind-altering drug being researched at this time. Many other medical professionals/ researchers had been exploring the effects of so-called traditional psychedelics such as LSD since the 1950s, most notably as a promising treatment for alcoholism and substance abuse disorders. A new model of therapy, psychedelic-assisted psychotherapy (PAP), began to emerge. The idea behind PAP was that psychedelics—when administered alongside psychotherapy—could help patients view their conditions from a fresh perspective, providing tremendous therapeutic benefit.

# PROHIBITION OF PSYCHEDELICS BEGINS

1966 didn't just mark the first year ketamine research was published. It also marked the beginning of a period in which the prohibition of psychedelics and the curtailment of research began in the United States. It was the year LSD was made illegal, a decision heavily influenced by Dr. Timothy Leary's sway over American youth.

A clinical psychologist at Harvard University, Dr. Timothy Leary is perhaps best known for founding the Harvard Psilocybin Project in 1960. Having experienced profound epiphanies from the use of magic mushrooms in Mexico, Leary became inspired to study the effects of psilocybin, the active ingredient in magic mushrooms.

Conducted between 1960 and 1962, the project tested the thera-peutic effects of psilocybin as well as LSD.

The therapeutic drug use in this project seemed to exert an over-whelmingly positive effect on subjects. Seventy-five percent of the subjects who participated in the project described their psilocybin experience as "very pleasant." Sixty-nine percent of participants reported experiencing a "marked broadening of awareness." A whopping 95 percent of subjects claimed their psilocybin sessions had "changed their lives for the better" (Weil 1963).

Leary's effect on popular culture was profound. He began urging American youths to use psychedelics like LSD when the Vietnam War was in full swing. The resulting effect? According to Ahmed Kabil in "The History of Psychedelics and Psychotherapy," young people told their parents they no longer believed in the central institutions undergirding American society and certainly did not want to fight in Vietnam. This, of course, raised alarm bells in the US government.

Leary was arrested 36 times during the 1960s and 1970s. His influence was so great that President Richard Nixon reportedly referred to him as the most dangerous man in America.

And so LSD was made illegal in the US in 1966, with the DEA and FDA immediately shutting down all psychedelic-inspired avenues of research in what would later become known as the "war on drugs." The decision was especially unusual given the emerging research pointing to the therapeutic value of these substances. Even US Senator Robert Kennedy questioned this decision, perhaps due to the fact that his wife, Ethel, had reportedly received LSD therapy (Reynolds 2018). Determined to investigate why psychedelic research was being halted, Kennedy launched a formal probe into the matter. According to Lauren Reynolds, he asked:

Why if [clinical LSD projects] were worthwhile six months ago, why aren't they worthwhile now? I think we have given too much emphasis and so much attention to the fact that it can be dangerous and that it can hurt an individual who uses it that perhaps to some extent we have lost sight of the fact that it can be very, very helpful in our society if used properly.

Kennedy's concerns, however, went unreplied to, and so research into psychedelics remained at a standstill.

# "THE BUDDY DRUG"

Despite sharing some properties with traditional psychedelics, ketamine somehow remained exempt from the DEA's war on drugs. In fact, the first preparation of ketamine approved by the FDA for human use, Ketalar, was approved in 1970 due to its high level of safety and immediate response time (Li and Vlisides 2016). These properties led to its initial use as a field anesthetic administered to soldiers during the Vietnam war. Ketamine quickly became integral to trauma and emergency/combat field medicine. It could be administered in a number of different ways, including via injection. Its effects were rapid and it demonstrated a better safety profile than PCP. In fact, administration was so simple that soldiers could even give ketamine to someone in need on the battlefield, earning it the moniker of "the buddy drug."

While ketamine was being used to tend to soldiers in the battlefield, its psychedelic counterparts back at home faced greater restriction. In the year 1970, Ketalar became FDA approved *and* President Nixon passed the Controlled Substances Act, rendering LSD and psilocybin as Schedule I drugs with "no currently accepted medical use and a high potential for abuse" (DEA 2020).

# THE BIRTH OF KETAMINE CULTURE

Rogue "medicinal chemists," however, were utilizing ketamine all over the globe. London researcher Karl Jansen, a member of the Royal College of Psychiatrists and a ketamine expert, notes in his book, *Ketamine: Dreams and Realities*:

> My interviews revealed that as early as 1967–1968 ketamine was already being used outside of the hospital and laboratory. The drug was being spread by some rogue "medicinal chemists" from Michigan out to the Florida coast under the names of "mean green" and "rockmesc." Ketamine has long been sold as something other than what it actually is, as the early name "rock mescaline" implies.

The underground ketamine movement was already afoot by the 1970s. Rogue chemists, as Jansen notes, sought to capitalize on ketamine's therapeutic potential under the radar, while other pioneers tested its effects firsthand. One such pioneer in the world of ketamine was Marcia Moore.

Moore was an American writer who was extremely interested in ketamine's therapeutic properties. She was also the wife of Dr. Howard Sunny Alltounian, an anesthesiologist. The two sought to uncover more about ketamine and did so by experimenting with the drug firsthand. Moore and Alltounian published their discoveries in a book called *Journeys into the Bright World* in 1978. Alltounian took on the role of recording and transcribing Moore's first-hand findings during their experiences. As such, the book presents highly detailed accounts describing the wide range of ketamine's psychological effects. She touches on a number of subjects in her narration, including ketamine's influence on music, spirituality, and the arts. Moore also asserted the theory that ketamine allowed subjects "to access internal dualistic sub-personalities that unconsciously affect one's daily choices" (Fork 2012).

Its use spurred by influential works like Moore and Alltounian's, ketamine began hitting the streets by the end of the '70s—and quickly grew to become a concern for the FDA.

Access to ketamine had previously been confined to use by health-care practitioners and soldiers during the Vietnam War. Ketamine, however, soon began slipping into the mainstream through raves and techno music. Rave culture had just begun to take shape in the United States in the '80s, and as it did, new forms of ketamine began popping up in the street drug market.

Recreational users could now purchase ketamine as a tablet, in a capsule, as a powder, or even in injectable form. The drug was often sold as "ecstasy" at the time to eager, unsuspecting rave goers. Many of these "dud pills" appeared in underground raves and clubs across the UK. These dud pills may or may not have contained small amounts of ketamine, but more often than not they contained a mixture of other drugs, including MDMA and methamphetamine.

Moore, incidentally, "disappeared without a trace" in January of 1979 (Vincent 2021). Her remains were found in a Seattle suburb in 1981. Authorities have yet to uncover any evidence of foul play (*New York Times* 1981).

# THE REVIVAL OF PSYCHEDELIC RESEARCH

Psychedelic advancements in research were effectively placed on a more than 20-year hiatus until the early '90s. Scientists at the time—

across Germany, the US, and Switzerland—quietly began to revive the movement.

Of particular note here were the studies conducted by John H. Krystal and his colleagues in the early 1990s. Krystal, a psychiatrist and professor at Yale, demonstrated that a single infusion of ketamine could produce "behaviors similar to the positive and negative symptoms of schizophrenia" in patients. These effects included changes in perception and impaired performance on tests of vigilance and verbal fluency, and "evoked symptoms similar to dissociative states" (Krystal 1994).

This discovery had two very distinct effects. The first is that it sparked interest in scientists who sought out to learn more about this curious drug. The second, of course, is that it prompted a new wave of concerns regarding ketamine's safety profile. Krystal addresses these concerns in his later work when he revisits the concept of what a safe subanesthetic dose (or a dose smaller than what is needed for anesthesia procedures) of ketamine should ideally be (Perry et al. 2006).

But as ketamine's reputation grew among the medical community, it was making waves in the public eye in a far different manner. Illegal use of ketamine in underground dance clubs grew until it entered the mainstream. Tales of ketamine abuse began to spread. The FDA reported that since 1992,

> More than 775 reports of ketamine diversion or abuse have been received by the DEA. More than 568 law enforcement reports described encounters of individuals who sold the drug, who had it in their possession, and/or were under its influence. Veterinary clinic burglaries which were directed at ketamine were described also. The balance of the reports were of ketamine abuse related hospital emergency

department visits. (US Department of Justice and Drug Enforcement Agency 1999)

Citing the widespread distribution, misuse, and abuse of ketamine, the spreading notoriety of ketamine as a party drug, and the use of Special K by teenagers and young adults, the United States federal government categorized ketamine as a Schedule III substance in 1999, temporarily halting additional research into its potential therapeutic uses (Hendrix 2019) and recreational use.

---

## A BRIEF NOTE ON DRUG SCHEDULING

Just what distinguishes a Schedule III drug from a Schedule I drug, anyway? Here's a quick primer on the DEA's drug classification system.

**Schedule I:** These are substances with "no currently accepted medical use and a high potential for abuse." A few drugs in this category include heroin, LSD, and ecstasy.

**Schedule II:** These drugs are categorized by their high potential for abuse, with use that may lead to severe psychological or physiological dependency. Some examples of drugs in this category include cocaine, Vicodin, and oxycondone.

**Schedule III:** These drugs contain a moderate to low potential for dependence—less so than Schedule I and II drugs, but more so than Schedule IV drugs. Anabolic steroids and testosterone are some notable Schedule III drugs.

**Schedule IV:** Substances with a low potential for dependency and abuse fall into this category. These include drugs such as Valium, Xanax, and Ambien.

**Schedule V:** These are drugs with a with low potential for abuse that contain limited quantities of certain narcotics. Many of these drugs are used for analgesic, antidiarrheal, and antitussive purposes. A few of these substances include cough preparations with less than 200 milligrams of codeine.

(Drug Enforcement Administration 2018)

- - - - - - - - - - - - - - - - - - - - - - - - - - - - - - - - -

Ketamine became a Schedule III nonnarcotic substance under the Controlled Substances Act.

Scientists, however, were not so easily deterred. Medical professionals in the early 2000s started noticing ketamine exhibited fascinating properties with respect to depression. Krystal and his team at Yale School of Medicine published the first randomized trial demonstrating ketamine's effects in 2000 (Krystal et al. 2000). These researchers discovered that a single subanesthetic dose, rapidly improved depressive symptoms. This was evidenced via significant reductions in the Hamilton Depression Rating Scale, the most widely used clinician-administered depression assessment scale.

Several small randomized controlled trials beginning around this time served to reinforce this discovery (McElvery 2022).

In 2006, the National Institute of Mental Health reported that a single intravenous dose of ketamine had rapid antidepressant effects. This led medical providers to begin prescribing the drug off-label, particularly for patients with major depressive disorder (MDD) and other psychiatric conditions.

Meanwhile, across the pond in the UK, ketamine had become a poignant problem. In 2005, the *Guardian* released an article titled "Ketamine Made Illegal After Health Concerns," describing the drug as "a horse tranquilizer...rocketing in the underground club scene." By January of the following year, ketamine was made illegal for medical and recreational use in the United Kingdom.

# SPRAVATO: A NEW MIRACLE DRUG?

Ketamine was first patented in Belgium in 1963 (Dong et al. 2015). Its patent in the United States expired in 2002, leading enterprising pharmaceutical brands to scheme a way to capitalize on the drug (Goldhill 2020). Janssen Pharmaceuticals, a subsidiary of Johnson & Johnson (J&J), began searching for ways to market a unique version of the drug they could patent. They did so by creating esketamine, which they patented as Spravato.

Enantiomers are compounds that share the same molecular formula but are mirror images of each other. Ketamine is a racemic molecule with two enantiomers, S-ketamine and R-ketamine. A racemic compound is one which contains equal amounts of each enantiomer.

Since ketamine had been on the market for so long, it wasn't possible to patent its racemic mixture. In order to create a new molecule they could patent, Janssen split up racemic ketamine into its two parts, S-ketamine and R-ketamine. They took the isolated esketamine molecule and marketed it as Spravato, a spray-based drug geared toward patients with depression.

By 2013, Janssen Pharmaceutical had already filed a patent for esketamine, an act that launched a new wave of funded research on the drug (Singh and Caers 2023).

## CONTROVERSY

I have not yet uncovered (though I would be extremely interested to know) how much of the subsequent research emerging in this time period was funded by J&J, whether directly or indirectly. I'd venture to guess J&J's mark on ketamine research extends far beyond what we'd hope for. This is deeply concerning in a number of ways, to say the least. The first concern is that J&J can pay for a drug to be fast-tracked to FDA approval despite a lack of evidence suggesting the drug has been well tested and safe for humans. Other concerns include a fear of inherent bias in the research conducted on ketamine; after all, if J&J is paying, they're going to want the results to skew positively in their favor. This desire may also downplay any potential negative side effects of the drug, or minimalize any contraindications to allow greater drug access for higher capital gains. As such we have no way to truly know the extent to which J&J has influenced ketamine research and findings. For instance, as I was researching for this book, I found this note in an article about ketamine published by *Smithsonian Magazine* in 2022:

"Editor's note: Janssen Pharmaceuticals, the maker of Spravato, is a current advertiser with *Smithsonian Magazine*. The company did not have influence over or provide any direction in the editorial process, including this story."

Spravato was the first new drug approved for the treatment of severe depression in nearly three decades (Kaiser Health News 2019). It may have been hailed as a "miracle drug" by some, but the medical community at large did not celebrate its arrival. In fact, many were aghast to learn how Janssen Pharmaceuticals had senselessly split up ketamine for profit's sake. While the research is still in progress, many medical professionals asserted that racemic ketamine provided the most therapeutic benefit. Others pointed to the fact that mouse studies have shown the R-ketamine isomer to be "more potent and with less side effects than the S(+) isomer" (Zhang et al. 2014). Critics also alleged that Janssen's evidence in favor of Spravato "provided the FDA at best modest evidence it worked and then only in limited trials" (Huetteman and Kaiser Health News 2019). No information was presented regarding Spravato's long-term use or side effects beyond a 60-week period. Many cited unfair play, pointing to pharmaceutical companies that took advantage of FDA processes to quickly bring lucrative drugs to market.

According to an article published in *VICE*, physicians declared the new drug to be a rip-off, citing serious concerns Janssen Pharmaceuticals failed to address.

Esketamine was found to be no better than placebo in two out of the three short-term studies submitted to the FDA for approval. It was also found to be "unwieldy" to manage and carried a number of significant potential side effects. Most concerning of all was the fact that J&J's esketamine was *not even tested against racemic ketamine,* likely due to the fear that esketamine might perform more poorly than the racemic version (Oberhaus 2017).

The new drug, incidentally, came with a $900 per dose price tag (Silverman 2019). Racemic ketamine, however, is readily available for a fraction of the price.

"The biggest problem at hand is not the drug itself," continues Marco Ramos and his colleagues in a 2019 *VICE* article. "It's the fact that instead of representing a revolution in mental health treatment, as it has been touted to do, Esketamine [Spravato] is…just a way for pharmaceutical company Johnson & Johnson to make a significant profit off gullible insurance companies and vulnerable patients."

While the drug was still only legal for medical use, ketamine clinics began popping up around the country around this time. One of the first clinics, NY Ketamine Infusions, was opened by a Harvard-trained anesthesiologist, Glen Brooks, in 2012. Another notable provider, Ketamine Clinics Los Angeles, opened its doors to the world in 2014.

The FDA approved the use of Spravato in 2019 for treatment-resistant depression in adults, following up in August of that year with a second ruling allowing doctors to prescribe the drug for adults with imminent suicide risk. These decisions would inspire the launch of telehealth ketamine treatments in which patients could receive ketamine therapy at home, virtually revolutionizing the field overnight.

## ETHICAL CONCERNS: IS SPRAVATO THE ANSWER?

In my experience as a patient, racemic ketamine has been much harder to access than Spravato. When I initially sought out racemic ketamine, I went through my mental health-care provider's list of psychiatrists and called them one by one to ask if they would prescribe racemic ketamine.

To my complete amazement, many of them were unwilling to do so. Some cited reasons as simple as not being aware of ketamine's off-label use for conditions such as depression. In fact, most of the providers I spoke with were very hesitant to prescribe ketamine due to a lack of experience with racemic ketamine.

The providers I did speak with who had treated patients with ketamine had only done so with Spravato. I asked why this was the case and was told the reason behind this was that there were few guidelines detailing how physicians could prescribe ketamine for off-label use.

The term "off-label" refers to using a drug in a context outside of its originally intended application. In this case, since ketamine is primarily a drug used in surgery, any use of it to treat other conditions such as depression would be considered off label.

Racemic ketamine didn't have a list of guidelines for off-label use that was widely available for physicians. Therefore most psychiatrists opted for Spravato instead, which has extensive documentation outlining potential uses available, courtesy of J&J. This then created a system in which psychiatrists opted for Spravato, not because it was necessarily the most *effective* option available for their patients, but because it was the most familiar type of ketamine available to them.

This system has sinister implications—chiefly, that both J&J and psychiatrists are touting esketamine (Spravato) as a "revolutionary" drug when it may in fact be less effective than racemic ketamine. In doing so, access to racemic ketamine, which is far cheaper than Spravato, dwindles as patients are forced to pay hundreds for the more commonly available Spravato.

# DRUG EFFICIENCY: ESKETAMINE VS RACEMIC KETAMINE

Ketamine is also classified as an entheogenic substance. Entheogens are substances categorized by their ability to inspire feelings of heightened empathy, love, and joy along with alterations in perception. Entheogens such as cannabis, peyote, and psilocybin mushrooms are also typically used for spiritual and therapeutic purposes.

Research indicates that certain entheogens such as cannabis are therapeutically more effective when consumed as a whole plant extract. In the cannabis world, the term "full spectrum" means a solution contains all of a plant's various cannabinoids like THC, along with other substances like terpenes and flavonoids.

While more research is still needed to fully investigate, we do know that cannabis extracts that utilize only one part of the plant— known as isolates—are only effective up until a certain point. After that point you could continue to administer more isolate, but you won't see any additional therapeutic effect.

Full-spectrum (whole plant) extracts, on the other hand, do not demonstrate this stopping-off effect. They demonstrate far greater therapeutic efficiency than isolates alone. In other words, whole plant extracts are far more potent than their isolated components. We can think of esketamine as an isolate, a compound that does not utilize the full substance in its final formulation. Since access to ketamine has been so tightly regulated for so long, we cannot say it behaves the way cannabis does with absolute certainty. However, ketamine is also classified as an entheogenic substance, which suggests some commonalities may exist between the two. Cannabis also acts on NMDA receptors, which are the main receptor sites targeted by ketamine.

Unfortunately, research has not yet provided us with a well-designed trial comparing the efficacy of racemic ketamine to esketamine alone. We do, however, have some research that corroborates the idea that "whole extract," or racemic ketamine, is more effective than esketamine alone.

One study published in the 2016 edition of the *American Journal of Psychiatry* suggests that two or three weekly intravenous administrations of racemic ketamine may be superior to eskatamine co-initiated with another antidepressant (Singh et al. 2016). This finding, however, does not take examine esketamine administered on its own; the presence of the antidepressant administered with esketamine undoubtedly exerts an effect that isn't measured here. This poses another concern into the efficacy of esketamine: much of the available data documenting its therapeutic effect focuses on subjects who are taking antidepressants in addition to esketamine.

# ESKETAMINE SAFETY CONCERNS

In a 2019 editorial written by Dr. Alan Schatzberg in the *American Journal of Psychiatry*, Schatzberg raised concerns associated with esketamine's rising popularity. To my horror, he noted that six deaths had occurred in esketamine's clinical trial program, which only had 197 subjects enrolled. Adding to my dread was the fact that this information seemed to be kept well-hidden, as I had never come across information about these deaths until nearly completing this book. Three of the deaths were suicides. There were no suicides in the control group (Schatzberg 2019).

Part of what makes this information so terrifying is the fact that several patients who committed suicide *appeared* to be improving in their depression scores—on paper, that is.

To what lengths had someone gone to keep this information quiet? How could the FDA possibly approve such a drug?

Schatzberg also cited the fact that the rate of patient relapse in the esketamine trial was 40 percent three to four months after treatment. Imagine that: even with an antidepressant added on, Spravato still didn't seem to be very effective. If that isn't indication on its own that Spravato doesn't work, I don't know what is. If anything, the more I learn about this drug, the more anxious I feel about it being the most common version of ketamine available to patients.

# THE CURIOUS CASE OF ESKETAMINE'S FDA APPROVAL

I haven't tried Spravato firsthand, so I cannot personally vouch for its use or efficacy. However, everything I've learned about this drug seems to imply it was fast-tracked through the FDA and approved without adequate testing. Spravato was never compared against racemic ketamine, for starters, *and* the drug was only evaluated over a short period. Conventional drugs must typically show testing on subjects over a long enough period to demonstrate that the long-term safety effects and potential contraindications of a drug have been fully evaluated. In the FDA's case, the standard drug review, aka the drug approval process for drugs that offer minor improvements over existing therapies, is set at ten months. The priority review status given to drugs that offer major improvements over conventional options is set at six months (Center for Drug Evaluation and Research 2019).

The efficacy of Spravato was evaluated in three short-term (four-week) clinical trials and one longer-term maintenance-of-effect trial. Did I forget to mention that all of the patients in these studies started—and continued—a new oral antidepressant throughout the trials (Daly et al. 2019)?

At this point you might very reasonably be wondering how on earth a drug with minimal testing could possibly get approved.

COVID-19 had hit Americans hard, especially with respect to depression. Rates of depression skyrocketed from 8.5 percent prepandemic to 27.8 percent. Additional research from Boston's University School of Public Health reveals that these elevated rates of depression persisted and have even worsened into 2021, climbing to 32.8 percent (McKoy 2021).

In an effort to combat rising rates of depression, the FDA implemented a number of new regulatory changes. These include increased access to telehealth services, which in turn led to more off-label, unsupervised use of the drug (Backman 2023).

Meanwhile Johnson & Johnson and the FDA continued to promote Spravato to desperate patients at home.

Emmarie Huetteman, associate Washington editor at Kaiser Health News, sums it up best, writing:

> Esketamine's trajectory to approval shows—step by step—how drugmakers can take advantage of shortcuts in the FDA process with the agency's blessing and maneuver through safety and efficacy reviews to bring a lucrative drug to market.

Esketamine is a glaring example of how the FDA, an agency designed to protect the American people, has taken advantage of the very people it was meant to protect for financial gain.

Incidentally, a meta-analysis published in 2020 found IV ketamine to be more efficacious than intranasal esketamine (Spravato) for the treatment of depression (Bahji et al. 2020). A 2021 study aiming to investigate the long-term efficacy of intranasal esketamine (Spravato) in treatment-resistant major depression even concluded that "currently, the level of proof of Esketamine efficacy in long-term treatment-resistant treatment remains low" (Capuzzi et al. 2021).

# Chapter 2

# WHAT IS KETAMINE & HOW DOES IT WORK?

Today ketamine is often colloquially referred to as a horse tranquilizer. This was undoubtedly influenced by the 2005 *Guardian* article. But is ketamine actually a tranquilizer? Just what exactly is this strange substance, anyway?

Now that we've gone over the history of this fascinating drug, we're going to examine this unique compound in closer detail. How does ketamine work and produce its distinct effects? What do these effects entail?

Ketamine, as you now know, is a synthetic, man-made drug often associated with tranquilizing effects.

"One misconception is that ketamine is meant for horses," says Charles Patti, Chief Brand Officer for MY Self Wellness (https://myselfwellness.center), a ketamine therapy program operating in Florida.

Ketamine *is* a commonly used anesthetic in the animal world—but that's largely due to the fact that it "has a safety profile so outstanding that it's used on animals and is the number one choice for pediatric sedation for children 18 months and older," says Patti. It's most commonly used in ER settings to immobilize children for surgeries that may involve painful procedures or to minimize movement in children as they are administered treatment. Intravenous and intramuscular (IM) are the most common administration routes. An initial IV dose is typically 1–1.5 milligrams per kilogram over 1–2 minutes immediately before the procedure, and subsequent incremental dose(s) of 0.25-0.5 mg/kg every 10 minutes until the procedure is complete as needed. Intramuscular dosing uses an initial dose of 4 milligrams per kilogram with a maximum of 6 milligrams per kilogram ("Clinical Practice Guidelines: Ketamine Use for Procedural Sedation" 2021).

That does not mean, however, that ketamine isn't suitable for human treatment.

Ketamine has been a staple of veterinary medicine and is still commonly used in pediatric practice today. While ketamine has many useful clinical applications for both animals and humans, its label as an animal tranquilizer is problematic for a number of reasons. Dubbing the drug an animal tranquilizer conjures up fearful associations, giving ketamine an unfortunate reputation it has been saddled with for decades.

In a 2008 study, Karenza Moore and Fiona Measham of the University of Lancaster investigated the motivations behind ketamine use in England. The two uncovered a wealth of insight into how people commonly viewed ketamine. One participant described the phenomenon as "embarrassing, cos people that don't understand it are like 'that is a horse tranquiliser'. It's like someone starting taking dog worming tablets, why would you do that? Some people are just like 'why?'" (Moore 2008).

It's most likely that the animal tranquilizer association was picked up by journalists after hearing about the veterinary clinics that had been robbed (see the FDA's comments regarding ketamine abuse in "The Revival of Psychedelic Research" section in chapter 1 for more). The more drastic the headline, the greater the sales. And so it goes.

"Tranquilizer" is a term used to describe a broad category of drugs whose effects include relaxation, sedation, muscle relaxation, and anti-agitation. While ketamine technically can fall under this category, these effects only occur with large doses, doses far greater than recreational or therapeutic doses.

Ketamine is an anesthetic drug. We briefly touched on anesthetic drugs in chapter 1, noting how they are employed to prevent the sensation of pain and to decrease awareness in surgical patients.

Ketamine, however, isn't your average, run-of-the-mill anesthetic due to its unique dissociative properties.

# DISSOCIATION, EXPLAINED

The term "dissociative anesthesia'" was coined specifically to describe ketamine's unique effects on patients. But just what does this phenomenon entail, exactly?

Despite not being a member of the "traditional" hallucinogen family (LSD, DMT, psilocybin), ketamine's unique dissociative properties imbue it with psychedelic-like, or psychotomimetic effects (Bowdle et al. 1998). Patients taking ketamine can appear to be awake but be unresponsive to stimuli. At low concentrations, they might hallucinate, experience out-of-body sensations, or experience other cognitive distortions that could impact mood and perception of reality.

Intense analgesia, or a drastic loss of pain sensation, is coupled with increased sympathetic activity, or activation of the body's "rest" state. Curiously enough, some patients also experience a state of euphoria at this time.

A 2006 study described ketamine as producing four main psychological effects:

1. a feeling of intoxication, comparable to the effects of other anesthetics and sedatives;

2. perceptual alterations in visual, auditory, and somatosensory domains concomitant with symptoms of depersonalization or derealization;

3. referential ideas and delusions, often of misinterpretation and thought disorder; and

4. negative symptoms such as poverty of speech (also known as laconic speech, a condition characterized by a lack of speaking). (Pomarol-Clotet et al. 2006)

Depersonalization is defined as the sensation of feeling as though you are observing your body externally. It can also refer to the feeling that things around you aren't quite real, or can be experienced as a combination of the two. Derealization is a state of feeling detached from your surroundings. These sensations coupled together produce the unique sensation known as dissociation.

Clinical professionals have described these unusual, hypnotic-like states as those in which patients were physically present but mentally "not there."

Interestingly enough, ketamine—unlike most gaseous anesthetics—does not cause a decrease in heart or respiratory rate (Corssen and Domino 1966). This has been a huge advancement in the medical field since respiratory depression, a decrease in respiratory rate, is commonly seen in patients recovering from surgery and anesthesia due to the residual effects of anesthetic agents. Respiratory

THE KETAMINE HANDBOOK

depression is a potentially life-threatening condition in which respiration, or breathing rate, does not provide adequate air flow. Ketamine's effects are also unique in the sense they are very much dose-dependent. Subanesthetic doses, or doses smaller than those needed to sedate patients, produce ketamine's characteristic psychotomimetic properties, while larger doses lead to sedation and unconsciousness (Krystal et al. 2000).

# MECHANISM OF ACTION

Despite ketamine's promising therapeutic potential, no one is quite sure how ketamine works.

We're not *totally* clueless, though. Scientists have a few hypotheses that attempt to explain ketamine's unique mechanism of action. The leading theory at the moment postulates that ketamine acts in such a manner so as to improve neuroplasticity. Neuroplasticity refers to the brain's ability to adapt in response to external situations such as traumatic injury. It's accomplished through the creation of new neural pathways in the brain. These new neural pathways can also help us break free of old habits and create new, more beneficial patterns that allow us to change for the better.

How does ketamine help create this neuroplastic state? Time to dive into the delicious nitty gritty of it all.

## GABA AND GLUTAMATE

If ketamine is the hero of this story (and trust me, it is), then gamma-aminobutyric acid (GABA) and glutamate are our leading ladies. Allow me to explain.

Leading theories point to ketamine's ability to affect GABA and glutamate receptors. GABA and glutamate are both neurotransmitters, chemical messengers designed to carry signals between nerve cells (neurons). Neurotransmitters carry nerve impulses by traveling across synapses, or junctions between neurons.

Each nerve cell has a unique membrane with receptors on it. Chemical messengers and molecules can interact with these receptors in a number of ways, including the following.

## MAINTAINING BALANCE: EXCITATORY VS INHIBITORY

Glutamate and GABA regulate our sympathetic and parasympathetic nervous system responses, otherwise known as the "fight or flight" and "rest and digest" states. Sympathetic function alerts the body to incoming threats, helping prepare it for a state of battle ("fight") in a number of ways. These include the release of adrenaline, prompting increased heart rate and the widening of bronchial passages to get more oxygen in. The primary neurotransmitter involved in this process is glutamate, an excitatory neurotransmitter. Glutamate's healthy function is imperative to proper cell functioning. It's involved in a number of processes pertaining to learning and memory, including neurodevelopment, neurocognitive (memory learning), and neurotrophic (nerve growth differentiation, maintenance) function (Mandal et al. 2019). Studies also show that patients with MDD have decreased hippocampal volume, an area of the brain responsible for memory function. This has been linked to glutamate dysregulation and treatment resistance to traditional antidepressants (Abdallah et al. 2022).

The parasympathetic nervous system, on the other hand, promotes a state of rest following sympathetic activation. Its primary function is to conserve energy that is later used to regulate body functions such as urination and digestion. In the central nervous system, GABA is the principal inhibitory neurotransmitter. It decreases stimulation of neurons, effectively blocking nerve transmission, and is

THE KETAMINE HANDBOOK

known to produce a relaxing or calming feeling. It's implicated in a host of other functions, including sleep regulation, mood, memory, circadian rhythms, and even perception of pain. GABAergic neurons also regulate brain circuits in the amygdala, the brain's "fear" center, to modulate stress and anxiety responses.

"There's a homeostasis between glutamate and GABA, and when you're anxious or depressed or have a dependency on a substance, that balance is off," says Dr. Abid Nazeer, a psychiatrist with double board certifications in both psychiatry and addiction medicine. While healthy glutamate functioning is a vital part of a functioning nervous system, it can go haywire. Too much glutamate can excite cells to their death, a process known as neurotoxicity. This process of cell death via cellular cytotoxicity actually points us to one of the major leading theories behind depression.

## DEPRESSION, GABA, AND GLUTAMATE

Major depressive disorder (MDD) is associated with a few distinct differences in the brain, especially in two critical areas: the prefrontal cortex (PFC) and hippocampus of the brain. When a receptor site is stimulated too often our bodies will do everything they can to maintain homeostasis.

Let's say you're exposed to an acute threat—something in front of you is trying to attack you!—and the sympathetic nervous system is activated into "fight" mode (an excitatory state). This activation releases a wave of neurotransmitters and hormones, such as adrenaline, into the bloodstream, helping you fight off the threat. In this way, acute stress can actually promote synaptic survival and strength, leading to the creation of behaviorally adaptive responses (e.g., enhanced working memory) (Abdallah et al. 2017).

However, in the case of chronic stressors, or when a person is continually exposed to a threatening environment, the sympathetic nervous system is constantly stimulated. Too much stimulation, as we learned above, can excite neuronal cells to their death, leading them to atrophy, a state we call excitotoxicity. This excitotoxicity leads to dysfunctions in the strength between neurons (synaptic strength) and reduced dendritic branching, especially within the PFC (Abdallah et al. 2022). Dendrites are the long, spindly arms of neurons that receive communication from other cells. Their "branches" are what carry nerve impulses over from one neuron to the next. When these arms are overstimulated, they degrade in a way so that they are able to carry less information from cell to cell.

In an attempt to regulate all of this excitatory stimulation, our bodies can then downregulate, or attempt to utilize less of its resources at that given area. Downregulation is accomplished by making cells less responsive to a chemical agent. In glutamate's case, down-regulation is mediated by inflammatory cytokines (compounds that denote the presence of inflammation) and neurotrophins such as brain-derived neurotrophic factor (BDNF). Downregulation can also cause negative structural changes to the synapses them-selves, reducing synaptic strength, dendritic spine density, and overall dendritic branching within the PFC (Abdallah et al. 2022). In short, connectivity between certain regions of the brain becomes damaged or diminished.

The abnormalities we see in the brains of patients with MDD, then, are believed to be the result of downregulation due to excitotox-icity, or excessive chronic stimulation (Abdallah et al. 2015). In an attempt to maintain balance, our bodies can remain stuck in this downregulated state in which cells are less responsive. The state of chronic downregulation is thought to manifest as depression.

So what does all of this have to do with ketamine again? Read on for answers.

# UNDERSTANDING KETAMINE'S MECHANISM OF ACTION

Remember how we said no one is quite sure how ketamine works? That may be the case, but a number of leading hypotheses point to the ways ketamine interacts with GABAergic neurons and glutamate as one of its primary mechanisms of action. At this point in time, the release of glutamate is believed to be the main mechanism by which ketamine exerts its rapid antidepressant properties.

"It is likely that the glutamate surge, prefrontal synaptogenesis, and prefrontal connectivity are implicated in ketamine's psychiatric effects for non-depressive disorders, but these ideas are largely hypothetical at present" (Abdallah et al. 2022).

Let's talk about this glutamate surge a little bit.

## WAKING UP DORMANT NEURAL PATHWAYS

One type of receptor found at excitatory synapses is the N-methyl-D-aspartate (NMDA) receptor. NMDA receptors play a vital role in cell plasticity, learning, memory formation, and neuroplasticity. These receptors open and close in response to glutamate via voltage-gated ion channels.

Ketamine, however, is an NMDA receptor antagonist, meaning it interacts with this receptor in two curious ways:

**1.** as an open channel blocker, attaching to the receptor site and binding to it in such a way so that it prevents the passage of cations (positively charged ions), and

**2.** as an allosteric modulator, a substance which reduces the amount of time and frequency the channel is open.

Ketamine's rapid antidepressant effects are, at this time, largely believed to be the result of its ability to block NMDA receptor function. When ketamine is introduced into the system, it blocks NMDA receptors located on GABAergic neurons. This blockade, in turn, prompts a surge of glutamate to be released into the brain's PFC.

"Ketamine can bring about rapid improvements in mood by restoring glutamate signaling," says Dr. Robison, a board-certified psychiatrist and chief medical officer for Numinus, a mental health care company that provides patients with access to safe, evidence-based psychedelic-assisted therapies. "I like to compare this to waking up dormant neuronal pathways like you're jump starting a car battery, so these pathways can communicate more freely."

When I used to get *really* depressed, I'd stay at home…for a loooong time. Sometimes I wouldn't emerge from my hidey-hole for weeks. I'd lay in there cooped up, lacking the energy to change my clothes or go outside for days at a time. Despite spending my days doing virtually nothing, I felt utterly drained of energy. Completing a basic task seemed to require a Herculean effort—until ketamine came in, that is, and WOKE ME UP.

With each dose of ketamine, I found that my desire to do things returned in full force. My anhedonia, or lack of motivation to do anything, vanished. I'd often bolt up from the couch, surprised as though someone else was puppeting me, and find myself walking outside seconds later. It was almost as though the part of me that truly wanted to *live* could finally do so without interruption. I became interested in things again—so very alive.

That feeling, in part, is likely due to a ketamine-induced glutamate surge. Release of extra glutamate activates a number of cell-signaling pathways including those involving BDNF.

BDNF is a key molecule involved in neuron survival and growth, aka neuroplasticity processes. It's also heavily implicated in depression. Researchers are able to trigger depressive symptoms in animals by reducing BDNF. Conversely, we're also able to see that increasing BDNF produces antidepressant-like effects in rodents (Abdallah et al. 2022). It's also worth noting that PFC abnormalities are implicated in a number of psychiatric conditions, including bipolar disorder, PTSD, and ADHD (Carrion et al. 2009; Gamo and Arnsten 2011).

# OPENING THE WINDOW OF NEUROPLASTICITY

The release of BDNF promotes synaptogenesis, or the creation of new synaptic pathways. In fact, animal studies have already shown that ketamine administration promotes the rapid development of new synapses in the medial prefrontal cortex (mPFC) area (Li et al. 2010). Positron emission tomography (PET) studies also show low-dose ketamine increases brain metabolism, especially within the PFC. Ketamine's antidepressant effect is also associated with increased connectivity between the caudate, a structure of the brain located near the thalamus, and several brain regions, including mPFC (Abdallah et al. 2022).

"This opens up what we call a window of neuroplasticity, which is an opportunity to do therapy more productively," continues Robison. "The treatment of many mental health conditions requires creating new neuronal pathways in the brain to help people learn new ways of coping and living. Ketamine is kind of like sprinkling Miracle-Gro on neurons, helping make new connections and strengthen others."

# NEW WAYS TO COPE AND LIVE

Make no mistake, ketamine is a wonder drug—but not in the way you might think. Ketamine isn't a miracle cure-all. Taking the drug on its own won't accomplish much in terms of your depression.

The way ketamine can radically help alleviate depression is when you consciously and deliberately choose to capitalize on its neuro-plastic properties.

Let's consider cigarette smokers for a moment (I used to smoke for a decade myself). Many smokers feel that their brains have become hardwired to crave their fix of nicotine whenever they're stressed. Years of smoking cigarettes primes a smoker's brain to associate nicotine with a reward. With this kind of pattern established, com-pulsive reinforcement begins to create grooves in the brain.

As a former addict and chain-smoker I'd often be restless when I couldn't get my hit. I'd focus on little else, counting the seconds 'til I was able to go out and relieve the discomfort of jonesing. But some part of me also felt helpless, trapped by my addiction, frustrated and forlorn. I hated that cigarettes had so much power over me; hated that they damaged my health and my wallet for damn sure, too. Despite wanting to quit, I felt powerless to do so. My mind felt stuck in a cycle: discomfort (craving a smoke) → desire to alleviate discomfort (smoking the cigarette) → leading to additional dis-comfort (irritated lungs, poor mood) that, of course, eventually led to the desire to alleviate my discomfort again (another cigarette). The grooves in my brain, the reward-seeking center I'd primed for years, felt like they were etched in so deeply I couldn't reshape my mind.

Many smokers I know feel the same way: trapped, wanting to escape but not knowing how.

In this instance, ketamine could tremendously benefit someone looking to quit. The administration of ketamine itself wouldn't necessarily kill your desire to smoke instantly. But it just might help you create new neural pathways outside of the pre-etched grooves in your brain, a new track you can choose to play. It might help inspire a train of thought in which you're able to be truly mindful without panic, a state of introspection Buddhists call "wise mind."

I was never able to access my wise mind state without ketamine; I was always too busy reacting to my emotions rather than observing, feeling, and processing them fully. Ketamine, however, allowed me to observe without judging or reacting. It helped my mind discover new insight into why I smoked and why I had those cravings. It also forced me to confront the ugly truth I kept trying to hide: that smoking cigarettes would eventually seriously damage my health. Sober, smokeless me ran and ran from this thought every time I lit up—but on ketamine I could not ignore it any longer.

I felt like I discovered another way of learning things. This new introspective state where I could observe without reacting, where I could sit with my thoughts without feeling terror, was a game changer in every sense of the word. It felt like uncovering a superpower. I felt more awake, like all of my brain could finally communicate with itself.

"When you are in a neuroplastic state, it's easier to be motivated," says Dr. Nazeer. "You get much more out of psychotherapy and behavioral changes, lifestyle changes, exercise, and optimizing your other medications and treatments. Everything else you do surrounding the ketamine is going to help ketamine's neuroplastic state have a longer-lasting benefit."

"Everything else you do" should certainly include diet, sleep, and exercise. It should also include psychotherapy with a trusted provider.

"Ketamine doesn't instantly eradicate psychopathologies or deeply ingrained patterns," says Dr. Reid Robison, a board-certified psychiatrist and chief medical officer for Numinus.

"It's most effective when it is used as a catalyst or facilitating agent for psychotherapy tailored to the individual's unique struggle."

And so in this way, if a person is already primed for growth, if a person is willing to *do the work* associated with unfucking themselves, then ketamine can be a life-changing tool. It can help you access new states of thinking, behaving, and doing that may not have occurred to you before; or even help you shed new perspective on a subject your brain has been stuck on. It's a tool best taken in conjunction with psychotherapy, a healthy diet, lots of delicious sleep, and the genuine desire to go out there and make a change.

# OTHER MECHANISMS OF ACTION

Ketamine's blockade of NMDA receptors triggers a glutamate surge, promoting synaptogenesis. Synaptogenesis entails new spine growth, improved spine density, and dendritic branching—all of which enhance neural connectivity. These effects are thought to reverse the negative effects of chronic stress and depression, particularly within the prefrontal cortex.

But the blockade of NMDA receptors isn't the only way ketamine interacts with our system. Ketamine has been shown to interact with a wide range of cellular processes. Researchers note that each system doesn't act on its own, but rather acts with the others as one integrated nervous system (Sleigh et al. 2014).

According to the study by Abdallah et al. (2022), "Although the presented model focused on the well-studied NMDA-based ketamine's pathways, other promising complementary mechanisms have been proposed and await supportive evidence."

Let's explore a few of these other systems.

# REWARD CENTER

"Giving ketamine is kind of like taking a fire extinguisher to the 'fire' of stress in the brain," says Robison.

The lateral habenula (LHb) is known as the "anti-reward center" in the brain. This region funnels information from the front and center of the brain to areas that produce neurotransmitters such as serotonin and dopamine (Ramanujan 2022).

Too much activity in the LHb prompts it to enter a rapid-fire "burst mode," turning off dopamine production. Research also indicates animals with depressive-like symptoms show increases in lateral habenula neuronal burst activity (Yang et al. 2018). Aberrant increases in LHb activity are also linked to "anhedonia, helplessness, excessive focus on negative experiences, and, hence, depressive symptomatology" (Gold and Kadriu 2019).

Ketamine has been found to rapidly turn off and reset "burst mode" in the lateral habenula—specifically, by "silencing" excessive NMDA receptor dependent burst firing in LHb (Cui et al. 2019). When it's reset, it can give the individual a break from their chronic state of stress or overwhelm.

"This can facilitate emotion processing and allow the individual to experience positive mood states, including pleasure and savoring," adds Robison.

# OPIOID RECEPTOR

Ketamine is also known to produce activation of endogenous opioid systems. Endogenous opioids are compounds our bodies naturally produce to help us manage pain.

Opioid systems play a central role in the treatment of affective disorders, or conditions characterized by their ability to impact the way we feel. Animal literature also supports the idea that opioids are implicated in depression (Williams et al. 2018)

Clinical evidence suggests that ketamine's ability to relieve pain may involve interactions between NMDA receptor antagonists and opioid receptors (Williams et al. 2018).

Interestingly enough, research has found that Naltrexone, a medication designed to help treat opioid or alcohol abuse, is found to reduce the effect of ketamine. Naltrexone is an opioid receptor antagonist that blocks the effects of opioids (Joseph et al. 2021). This further speaks to the idea that ketamine's effects are in part mediated by the opioid system.

# RELIEVING DEPRESSION AT THE SPEED OF SEROTONIN

Selective serotonin reuptake inhibitors (SSRIs) are the most commonly prescribed substances for depressed patients (Chu and Wadhwa 2021). These medications work by preventing the reuptake, or reabsorption of serotonin by neurons. One effect is more extracellular serotonin becomes available, which can provide a number of therapeutic benefits.

While ketamine isn't classified as an SSRI, it may still act on serotonin. Researchers have suggested that ketamine may be able to inhibit the reuptake of serotonin as one hypothesis for how ketamine might produce its painkilling effects (Martin et al. 1982). Interestingly enough, while both SSRIs and ketamine may be able to influence serotonin levels, the two act at drastically different speeds. SSRIs typically take a minimum of 7 to 14 days to begin to reduce symptoms. Many patients, however, do not see results until several weeks of treatment (usually 4 to 12 weeks) have elapsed (Mandal et al. 2019). SSRIs also come with a host of serious side effects, including nausea, weight gain, and sexual dysfunction. Ketamine, however, has shown antidepressant effects almost instantaneously after administration, with as little as one dose. Effects were noted "immediately after the administration of ketamine and sustained at the end of 1 month" (Ferguson 2001). Few serious side effects are reported in studies administering ketamine treatment for depression.

## NICOTINE RECEPTOR

The current prevailing NMDA receptor theory doesn't fully explain ketamine's mechanism of action in its entirety (Lester et al. 2015). Some scientists are proposing that ketamine's blockade of another receptor site may explain its unique properties—specifically, blockade of the $\alpha 7$ and $\alpha 3\beta 4$ nicotinic receptors (Moaddel et al. 2013). These nicotinic receptors respond to the neurotransmitter acetylcholine, the chief neurotransmitter of the parasympathetic nervous system. Researchers postulate that ketamine's inhibition of these receptor sites may contribute to its distinct effects.

While emerging research suggests that ketamine may exert therapeutic effects with respect to addictive behaviors such as problematic alcohol and drug use, more research is needed to determine ketamine's effect on smoking cessation.

# THE DEFAULT MODE NETWORK & EGO DEATH

The default mode network (DMN) refers to a set of regions in the brain that are active during passive moments such as daydreaming or sleeping. Reports of default network dysfunction are linked to a number of psychiatric conditions, including depression, Alzheimer's disease, schizophrenia, and autism. Too much activity within this network is associated with other conditions such as obsessive compulsive disorder (OCD) (Buckner 2013).

The DMN is a region that's also implicated in ideas of ego dissolution. Ego dissolution, also known as ego death, refers to the phenomenon in which a person can experience a loss of self-identity. Ego deaths are characterized by a "reduction in the self-referential awareness that defines normal waking consciousness" and "increasing feelings of unity with others' and one's surroundings" (Mason et al. 2020). Distortions of self-experience are also linked to glutamate function (Mason et al. 2020).

Losing your sense of self, as it turns out, can actually be a good thing.

Ego death is one of the most liberating and terrifying things that can happen to you (in my experience). You lose awareness of self. You forget who you are. You begin to feel as though you are not, in fact, a separate, individual entity, but rather as though you belong to something bigger—the source of life itself. Everything can feel interconnected. A deep sense of harmony pervades your bones as you become one with the universe.

After my ego death, I was a far happier person in every sense of the word. I felt connected to nature and the things around me in a way I never had before.

Ketamine is able to act on our brains in a way that reduces DMN activity.

In 2010, Sheline and her colleagues proposed that reducing connectivity of the DMN might play a critical role in reducing depression symptoms. This represents a new potential therapy to target affective disorders (Scheidegger et al. 2012).

Ketamine exerts a "shutting down" effect on the default mode network, says Adam Mitchell of My Self Wellness.

"This perceived 'ego death' may be instrumental for the restructuring a person undergoes as they better adjust to their same life after the ketamine experience," says Mitchell.

Ketamine's effect on DMN connectivity supports the hypothesis that effective antidepressant treatment involves making systemic alterations within neural networks, aka rewiring your brain.

Significant restructuring of the brain's structures and its connections suggests a new model for treating depression—in contrast to the one based on correcting "imbalances" in one neurotransmitter or another.

## TACKLING RUMINATION

Just as increased connectivity in the DMN is associated with psychiatric conditions such as OCD, it can also lead to the phenomenon of rumination, a type of cognition where your brain focuses on negative content obsessively. Rumination is also linked to a number of psychiatric states, including depression and OCD.

Ketamine can tackle rumination by creating a temporary interruption between the cortex and the limbic system in the brain, giving a time-out from the ordinary mind to a space where there is less rumination and more cognitive flexibility. This flexibility can potentially help someone move on from a bad habit, free themselves of addictions and ruminative thoughts, or even inspire true change via a state of mindful introspection.

"I like to compare the mind to a ski slope. All of your thoughts and actions travel down it, and ruts and grooves are made in the snow," begins Robison. He continues:

> They get deeper and deeper over time, and pretty soon, no matter where you start or even aim, you're likely to slip into those same ruts and end up in the same location over and over. Like a ski slope, our minds develop patterns and ruts and grooves as we navigate the world. Ketamine, however, is like a fresh coat of powder, providing a break from the everyday patterns and let[ting] the brain reset the ruts, so you get to choose the next set of tracks, and end up consciously arriving at new destinations.

Ketamine's effects aren't short-lived, either. Research shows that ketamine's antidepressant effects can remain for one to two weeks after administration (Abdallah et al. 2022).

The behavior and effects of ketamine vary greatly depending on a number of factors. Each ketamine enantiomer, for instance, has a different bioavailability rate and may act in differing manners under unique circumstances. Intravenous ketamine, for instance, has a very high bioavailability rate of around 93 percent to 98 percent. Intramuscular ketamine has similarly high bioavailability. Oral ketamine, however, can have bioavailability as low as 20 percent (Abdallah et al. 2017).

We briefly touched on the idea of enantiomers as compounds that share the same formula but are mirror images of one another. Let's explore the concept of enantiomers in a little more detail.

# ENANTIOMERS

A racemic compound is one which contains equal amounts of each enantiomer. Ketamine is a racemic molecule with two enantiomers, S-ketamine and R-ketamine.

The singular enantiomer S-ketamine is available as the drug Sparvato (esketamine) from Johnson & Johnson. The drug is the first of its kind to be FDA approved for the treatment of MDD (Major Depressive Disorder) in adults.

Understanding which enantiomer is a better candidate for therapeutic outcomes is a process that's still underway. Mitchell notes that research investigating the properties of each enantiomer with respect to treating certain conditions is still underway.

"Clear answers about which enantiomers may be more effective for specific issues (neuropathic pain vs PTSD, for instance) and what side effects each may be associated with await future research," says Mitchell (Mitchell 2022).

A 2021 meta-analysis found that racemic ketamine demonstrated a greater overall response than esketamine, with improved remission rates and lower dropouts seen in patients. Researchers concluded that intravenous (IV) ketamine "appears to be more efficacious than intranasal esketamine (Spravato) for the treatment of depression" (Bahji et al. 2021). More research, however, is still ultimately needed.

# R-KETAMINE VS S-KETAMINE

Each enantiomer has its own unique characteristics.

**Esketamine:**

○ has demonstrated three to four times greater anesthetic (painkilling) potency compared to the R(−) isomer (White et al. 1985);

○ often produces more visual sensations (Mitchell 2022); and

○ when used during surgery (intraoperative), can result in less cardiac stimulation, more rapid recovery, and fewer psychotomimetic side effects (Li and Vlisides 2016).

**The R-enantiomer:**

○ is associated with fewer gastrointestinal complications (Mitchell 2022);

○ has fewer side effects than esketamine in mice studies (Zhang et al. 2014);

○ has been shown to have "longer lasting antidepressant effects than (S)-ketamine in animal models of depression" (Bahji et al. 2021); and

○ may produce more bodily experiences and be absent of the visual components of S-enantiomer experiences (Mitchell 2022).

Researchers have postulated the idea that the (R) enantiomer may possibly confer some degree of "protective effects," especially with respect to psychotomimetic properties (Passie et al. 2021).

# METHODS OF KETAMINE ADMINISTRATION

Ketamine is soluble in both water and lipids and is available in a number of different forms. It can be insufflated as a powder, made into a lozenge for oral consumption, injected through an IV or intramuscularly (IM), or administered intranasally as Spravato. Ketamine can also be safely administered via subcutaneous, epidural, and rectal routes.

Much like the case with ketamine enantiomers, each method of administration comes with its own unique pros and cons. We'll outline a few of these below, paying special attention to bioavailability (rate of absorption), response time, and ease of administration.

## INHALATION/INSUFFLATION

Recreational ketamine is often snorted (insufflated) as white powder, with an average effect onset time of 5 to 30 minutes. And though ketamine can be consumed intranasally, insufflation is a bad idea for a number of reasons.

Snorting powders or other substances can damage the interior lining of your nasal cavity (mucosal membrane), which may impair your sense of smell. Use of unclean paraphernalia may be a risk factor for the onset of diseases, which can be transferred through nasal passages as well.

Last but not least, if you're buying drugs off the street, there's no way for you to actually know if what you're buying is, well, what you're hoping to buy. This leaves recreational users open to a slew of dangerous substances that may be sold as ketamine. *American Family Physician*, a peer-reviewed and evidence-based medical journal published by the American Academy of Family Physicians, notes that ketamine can be sold as "trail mixes" containing methamphetamine, cocaine, sildenafil citrate (Viagra), or heroin. Other ingredients found in seized recreational ketamine have included "amphetamine, benzocaine, cocaine, MDMA, methoxetamine,

paracetamol, piperazines, and synthetic cathinones (bath salts)"
(Corkery et al. 2021).

# INTRAVENOUS (IV)

The golden standard for therapeutic ketamine treatment today is IV administration, which rapidly attains maximum plasma concentrations. The effects of IV administration are felt nearly instantaneously, with a 100 percent bioavailability rate.

# INTRAMUSCULAR (IM)

The bioavailability of intramuscular ketamine is only slightly lower than IV ketamine at 93 percent. Peak plasma concentrations of the drug are achieved within 5 to 30 minutes of administration (Clements et al. 1982). One pharmacokinetic analysis reported a model-estimated bioavailability rate of IM ketamine administration in children at 41 percent (Hornik et al. 2018). This number is much lower than the bioavailability recorded in adults, possibly due to the lower ratio of muscle mass to body mass found in children than in adults.

# INTRANASAL (SPRAVATO)

Intranasal administration of ketamine has a much lower bioavailability than IV or IM routes at approximately 45 percent (Yanagihara et al. 2002). This amount can also vary widely depending on the amount absorbed through nasal mucosal passages and the amount swallowed. This method of administration is an attractive option for health-care providers as it is less invasive than using an IV, results in rapid absorption, and is exempt from first-pass hepatic metabolism (Malinovsky et al. 1996). First pass metabolism refers to the phenomenon in which a drug that is orally consumed is broken down through the digestive tract. Drugs that are exempt from this phenomenon have higher bioavailability rates, meaning more of the drug is absorbed for greater effect.

## ORAL CONSUMPTION/LOZENGE

Some medical providers may offer ketamine to patients in the form of a lozenge or tablet for oral consumption. This is due to the fact that oral dosing is a far more practical (and less invasive) administration route than IV delivery. Ketamine is also far easier to dose and maintain over time via oral administration.

Ketamine, however, exhibits a poor oral bioavailability rate of about 16 to 29 percent, with peak concentrations achieved 20 to 120 minutes following administration (Zanos et al. 2018). This is likely due to a phenomenon known as first pass metabolism, in which the digestive tract significantly reduces drug concentration before it can circulate freely (Zanos et al. 2018). First-pass metabolism is especially significant in the case of (S)-ketamine, with an oral bioavailability estimated to be between 8 and 11 percent (Zanos et al. 2018).

A 2013 study examining the effect of daily oral ketamine administration noted that the response rate of oral ketamine with respect to depression is similar to that of IV ketamine barring one key respect: response time.

> Unlike what was previously demonstrated, this effect [improvement in depressive symptoms] was more protracted (occurring over weeks rather than in minutes) and more sustained than found with IV infusions of ketamine (>2 weeks). A significant novel finding was a decrease in symptoms of anxiety in 100 percent of the cases. (Irwin et al. 2013).

In short, improvements in depressive symptoms with oral ketamine administration may be more sustained over time than with traditional IV administration. This discrepancy may be due to one of two factors: because there are fewer adverse effects for the oral administration of ketamine, or because of the differing bioavailability rates for intravenous and oral routes.

## RECTAL

Ketamine can be administered rectally. Intrarectal ketamine bioavailability is 25 to 30 percent (Zanos et al. 2019).

# SYSTEMIC EFFECT

Now that we have a better idea of the ways ketamine can be administered, let's dive into the drug's systemic effects across the body.

## CARDIOVASCULAR

Ketamine acts as a sympathomimetic agent at both subanesthetic (a dose smaller than what is needed to produce anesthesia) and anesthetic (surgical) doses. A sympathomimetic substance mimics the behavior of the sympathetic nervous system, which controls the body's fight-or-flight responses.

In this case, that looks like ketamine's ability to directly stimulate the central nervous system, which can result in increased heart rate and cardiac output (Corssen and Domino 1966). Ketamine can increase blood pressure as well, though levels have not reached hypertensive or dangerous levels in clinical settings (Liebe et al. 2017).

Therefore, patients with a history of high blood pressure or other heart concerns should consult with their doctors before using ketamine.

## PULMONARY

Opioid analgesics are often administered via IV during surgery to provide analgesia and supplement sedation for patients. While opioid analgesics are very useful during surgery, they come with quite the caveat: namely, they can depress ventilation, or the flow of air passing through the lungs (van der Schier et al. 2014). This is known as respiratory depression. Respiratory depression refers to the phenomenon in which the lungs are unable to function properly due to poor ventilation. This can result in an accumulation of carbon dioxide in the blood and reduced oxygen levels. In its most severe form, unrecognized respiratory depression can lead to respiratory arrest, in which breathing ceases entirely and death occurs within minutes. Respiratory depression due to opioids is known as opioid-induced respiratory depression (OIRD), a potentially life-threatening condition.

As we touched on earlier, part of what makes ketamine such a unique substance is the fact that it can function as an anesthetic agent without causing significant respiratory depression in patients (Corssen and Domino 1966).

Data gleaned from animal models suggests that low doses of ketamine might actually help stimulate respiration (Eikermann et al. 2012). This is consistent with the finding that one of ketamine's effects on the respiratory system is bronchodilation (Brown and Wagner 1999). Bronchodilators help facilitate breathing by relaxing muscles in the lungs, widening airways (bronchi). Upper-airway obstruction is common during anesthetic states as well as sleep.

It occurs when there's an occlusion (block) or narrowing of the airways leading to the lungs, and can be a life-threatening condition. Ketamine has been found to preserve upper airway reflexes during anesthesia (Eikermann et al. 2012).

# NEUROLOGICAL

Ketamine's effects may be neuroprotective for patients with brain trauma (Albanèse et al. 1997; Bar-Joseph et al. 2009). The possibility of increased neuroplasticity can have a number of different implications for trauma patients. One of these is a reduction in intracranial pressure, or of a growing feeling of pressure within the skull. This is a typical consequence of traumatic brain injuries. Ketamine is also an excellent drug to help keep trauma patients stable: it has a very favorable systemic hemodynamics profile that promotes pulmonary vasodilation and bronchodilation (Gregers et al. 2020). Hemodynamics refers to how blood flows through vessels. Vasodilation is the process by which blood vessels dilate, or expand. Bronchodilation, then, is when bronchi, or airways in the lungs, open and expand. In this instance, having a favorable hemodynamic profile means ketamine does not depress airway function, which is a potential side effect associated with other anesthetic drugs.

Research also suggests ketamine's unique properties may help protect patients from developing stress-induced disorders by improving individuals' ability to tolerate distress, also known as distress tolerance (Brachman et al. 2016).

# CLINICAL USES FOR KETAMINE: AT A GLANCE

Head spinning with facts? Check out a summary detailing ketamine's clinical uses in this nifty chart that follows.

## SUMMARY OF CLINICAL USES FOR KETAMINE

| ANESTHESIA | ANALGESIA AND SEDATION | PSYCHIATRY AND NEUROSCIENCE |
|---|---|---|
| **Advantageous settings:**<br>○ Hemodynamic instability<br>○ Pediatric patients<br>○ Uncooperative patients<br>○ Traumatic brain injury<br>○ Bronchospasm (a state in which muscles that line your airway tighten, narrowing airways and potentially resulting in a cough)<br>○ Battlefield/mass casualty | **Acute settings:**<br>○ Surgical procedures<br>○ Burns<br>○ Emergency department agitation/pain<br>○ Postoperative pain<br><br>**Chronic settings:**<br>○ Cancer pain<br>○ Complex regional pain syndrome<br>○ Phantom limb pain<br>○ Fibromyalgia<br>○ Ischemic pain<br>○ Migraines | **Emerging use:**<br>○ Depression<br>○ Suicidal ideation<br>○ PTSD<br>○ Schizophrenia<br>○ Consciousness |

*Source:* Li and Vlisides 2016

# Chapter 3

# THE THERAPEUTIC PROMISE OF KETAMINE

Now that you have an understanding of how ketamine works, I'll begin to summarize what we know about this compound so far— that is, the therapeutic promise of ketamine. What are our research findings regarding this substance? This chapter will include a brief history summarizing notable and especially promising clinical applications of ketamine, particularly with respect to treatment-resistant depression.

I know, I know. This is the part you've all been waiting for. Time to dive into ketamine's therapeutic applications, aka The Real Good Stuff™.

"One thing almost all psychiatrists can agree on," says psychiatry researcher Adam Kaplin, "is this: We need antidepressants that work more quickly and for more people" (Minkove 2019).

The World Health Organization states that depression is a leading cause of disability worldwide. It affects roughly 5 percent of the global adult population. Of those people, 7.4 million are American adults that suffer from treatment-resistant depression (World Health Organization). At its worst, depression can be fatal, with suicide as the fourth leading cause of death in 15- to 29-year-olds. Approximately 13 percent of Americans use antidepressants, with approximately 17 percent of the US population meeting diagnostic criteria for major depressive disorder (MDD). MDD is a chronic condition associated with "elevated risk of suicide, functional impairments, and a variety of socio-economic difficulties" (Abdallah et al. 2022).

The use of antidepressants more than doubled in economically developed countries between 2000 and 2015 (M. Stone et al. 2022). The hope was that an increase in these numbers would correspond to a decrease in depression rates. However that is decidedly not the case, as rates of depression have generally increased, particularly in younger age groups (Stone et al. 2018). Suicide rates, too, climbed, increasing more than 30 percent across 25 states between 1999 and 2016 (D. Stone et al. 2018). How and why can that be the case? Are conventional antidepressants—*gasp!*—not as effective as one might hope?

# THE TRUE EFFICACY OF ANTIDEPRESSANTS

The standard first-line treatment for depression in America is often a pharmacological one: namely, through the prescription of SSRIs. These drugs, however, pose a number of concerns that make their continued use for treatment questionable. These include serious side effects such as weight gain and sexual dysfunction as well as the risk of worsening depressive symptoms. In fact, emerging research has suggested the idea that many popular antidepressants may "induce a biological vulnerability, making people more likely to become depressed in the future." Much of the research we've uncovered in the last decade actually points to the idea that any relief SSRI patients may experience is largely due to the placebo effect (Kirsch 2014).

In 2014, Irving Kirsch, a lecturer in medicine at the Harvard Medical School, sought to investigate antidepressants and the placebo effect, which is when patients experience relief from symptoms just because they *feel* like they're receiving treatment, even though they are not. His team used the Freedom of Information Act to request data that pharmaceutical companies had sent to the FDA in the process of obtaining approval for six new antidepressants. Kirsch also noted that the six new antidepressants "accounted for the bulk of antidepressant prescriptions being written at the time." His paper, "Antidepressants and the Placebo Effect," revealed some not-so-surprising data:

1. Almost half of the clinical trials sponsored by the drug companies have not been published.

2. The results of the unpublished trials were known only to the drug companies and the FDA, and most of them failed to find a significant benefit of the drug over a placebo.

3. The results indicated that the placebo response was 82 percent of the response to these antidepressants.

*Eighty-two percent of patient response was due to the placebo effect!*

Kirsch also went on to explain that his analyses uncovered the mean difference between drug and placebo effects registered as less than two points on the HAM-D (1.8). The HAM-D is a scale that measures how depressed people are on a scale from 0 to 53 points. A six-point difference, Kirsch notes, "can be obtained just by changes in sleep patterns, with no change in any other symptom of depression."

In other words, the 1.8 difference observed was "small enough to be clinically insignificant."

"When published and unpublished data are combined, they fail to show a clinically significant advantage for antidepressant medication over inert placebo," Kirsch concludes.

Another one of Kirsch's studies, published in August 2022, discovered that about 15 percent of participants experienced a substantial antidepressant effect beyond placebo effect in clinical trials (Stone et al. 2022).

Patients who do manage to experience some degree of relief from the use of SSRIs, however, will need to wait: most SSRIs take at least two weeks before patients can feel effects. Access to therapy remains equally daunting, with many patients reporting having to wait up to six weeks before being able to access care, leaving those who need help the most in a vulnerable position (Brooks 2022). Even after SSRIs are prescribed, many patients will notice a "tapering off" effect in which treatments no longer remain effective after a certain time (Fava 2020).

# UNDERLYING CAUSES OF DEPRESSION IN THE US TODAY

Depression and chronic stress are prevalent, pressing concerns in the United States today. To better understand and address these conditions, it is important to examine the underlying biological, psychological, and social causes that contribute to their prevalence.

One of the most pervasive theories about depression is that it's caused by a neurotransmitter imbalance. This theory posits the idea that too much or too little of the four key neurotransmitters—serotonin, dopamine, norepinephrine and glutamate—creates dysfunctions in our systems that can result in anxiety or depression. While this idea was espoused for some time, emerging research suggests depression is caused by far more than neurotransmitter imbalance.

Genetics also play a large role. Certain individuals may be more prone to depression due to genetic, inherited factors. The presence of cytokines, for instance, is an inherited trait that can denote inflammatory conditions. High cytokine levels are also linked to a number of mental health conditions. Maladaptive or ruminative cognitive styles, too, might be genetic or inherited to a degree. Individuals with poor health, such as those with certain heart conditions, are also significantly more susceptible to experiencing a depressive episode.

We touched earlier on how COVID-19 tripled depression rates in America, with rates of depression continuing to worsen over time. Other social factors that play a role here include lack of access to health care as well as an inability to access specialized care. Long wait times, too, have been criticized as a fault in the American health-care system, contributing to the burden of disease.

# A CRISIS IN PSYCHIATRY

Troublesome though they may be, SSRIs hardly fail to encapsulate the full scope of the problem at hand. Drug research itself has been in decline in the development of new drugs since the 1970s. Research and development in psychopharmacology (the study of the use of medications in treating mental disorders) "came to a halt in 2010" (Schenberg 2018). Schenberg also notes that:

- "Approval of new molecular entities for psychiatric conditions by the US Food and Drug Administration (FDA) fell from 13 in 1996 to one in 2016, with 49 approved between 1996 and 2006 and 22 from 2007 to 2016."

- "In pharmacology conferences in the period [between 1996 and 2016] just about 5 percent of presentations were dedicated to human studies involving drugs with novel mechanisms of action."

The FDA was approving fewer drugs for mental disorders with each passing year. Data available on the efficacy of conventional antidepressants was not compelling: a 2022 meta-analysis characterizing the response of patients with major depressive disorder to antidepressants between 1979 and 2016 found only 15 percent of patients experienced a "substantial antidepressant effect" beyond a placebo. While some may feel a reduction in symptoms at two weeks, many antidepressants can take weeks, or even months, of continuous use before patients experience any symptom relief. Many patients taking antidepressants also report experiencing a number of serious side effects.

Meanwhile, the number of drugs created for the treatment of said mental disorders dwindled to a near halt.

In other words, those suffering from depression seemed to be out of luck. The need for novel drugs that could act quickly with minimal side effects, especially with respect to depression, has never been greater.

# IT'S A BIRD! IT'S A PLANE! IT'S... KETAMINE!

Given the stakes at hand, it's easy to see why Krystal's discovery in 2000 brought the medical community to its knees (see page 17). Ketamine's ability to relieve depression could be brought about in *as little as one administration*, with effects sustained for weeks after treatment. Cries of "wonder drug" spread across the land as scientists rejoiced. Hope! Hope!

Before we can dive into all of the exciting ketamine research being conducted today, let's take a moment to summarize ketamine's therapeutic properties to date.

# ANESTHETIC

As we noted earlier, ketamine was originally developed as an anesthetic agent. An anesthetic agent is a drug used during surgery that results in a loss of sensation, especially pain.

Ketamine is a popular anesthetic choice as it has been shown to exert analgesic (pain-killing) properties as well as its characteristic dissociative effects. It can be successfully used in medical or veterinary practice with minimal side effects and administered with ease.

The dissociative properties of ketamine coupled with its analgesic aspects make it an ideal drug for situations where people may be subjected to traumatic experiences. Dissociation can help a person launch into "autopilot" mode in which they are able to make decisions despite turbulent environments. Dissociation may also impact memory formation in such a way so as to protect the individual from recalling the worst aspects of their trauma.

## ANESTHETIC DOSING

An anesthetic dose of ketamine is used to sedate patients for surgical procedures. This is achieved in humans at a dose ranging from 1 to 2 milligrams of ketamine per kilogram of body weight (mg/kg) administered intravenously. Intramuscular dosage is generally 4 to 11 mg/kg. A 500 mg dose of oral ketamine would be required to achieve ketamine's anesthetic effects, or 8 to 15 mg/kg if administered rectally. Intranasal esketamine (Spravato) requires doses of 3 to 9 mg/kg to sedate patients (Zanos et al. 2018).

# ANALGESIC

One of the earliest reports documenting ketamine's analgesic properties was H. Weisman's report "Anesthesia for Pediatric Ophthalmology," published in 1971.

Intravenous ketamine is currently administered as an analgesic agent for the treatment of postoperative pain. Ketamine's ability to act as an analgesic agent has been compared to opioids; however ketamine does not depress the respiratory system in doing so.

## ANALGESIC DOSING

Subanesthetic doses of ketamine can provide sufficient analgesia at doses as little as 0.15 to 0.25 mg/kg, when administered via IV, or 0.5 to 1 mg/kg when administered intramuscularly to patients following acute trauma (Zanos et al. 2018).

Ketamine's analgesic effects have been observed at the following doses:

○ orally at the dose of 0.5 mg/kg twice per day for 15 days or at the single dose of 2 mg/kg;

○ intranasally at a dose ranging from 10 to 50 mg twice per day;

○ transdermally at the dose of 25 mg/mL released throughout a 24-hour period;

○ subcutaneous administration (injections made just under the skin) at a dose ranging from 0.05 to 0.15 mg/kg per hour for 7 days; and

○ rectally at the dose of 10 mg/kg (Zanos et al. 2018).

# MICRODOSING

Microdosing is a little more challenging to provide exact figures for. After all, individual responses to ketamine vary greatly depending on your unique body composition.

Twenty-five milligrams of ketamine via an oral lozenge is the starting dose I received when I began ketamine therapy. I was told this constituted the smallest possible therapeutic dose that could be detected by a person. So we can safely say microdoses begin at 25 mg or less.

As to when a microdose becomes a macro, that's going to be different for every person. It's likely that microdose amounts will be very similar to subanesthetic doses of ketamine, which can be felt at doses as little as 0.15 to 0.25 mg/kg.

# ANTIDEPRESSANT

If someone is suffering from acute mental health struggles, studies have shown ketamine can provide relief and even remission within one or two sessions. If someone is suicidal, they must consider this option, as it might be the quickest and most effective path toward getting out of the dark patterns and potentially saving their life.

—Dr. Zand, psychiatrist and founder of Better U & Anywhere Clinic (www.anywhereclinic.com)

Studies conducted in the early 2000s, particularly R. M. Berman's work (Berman et al. 2000) uncovered findings that a single dose of ketamine could provide lasting relief from depressive symptoms.

Ketamine also boasts a far more favorable safety profile and fewer side effects than traditional antidepressants. Meta-analysis examining ketamine across depression trials reveals a low frequency of serious adverse events. No significant adverse physical effects with low-dose ketamine have been reported in antidepressant trials to date (Mandal et al. 2019; see Short et al. 2018 for long-term reporting bias.). On the other hand, SSRIs come with a slew of serious side effects including weight gain, sexual dysfunction, and manifestation of other disorders such as tardive dyskinesia, a type of movement disorder.

A 2018 meta-analysis published in the *American Journal of Psychiatry* found that ketamine exerted rapid antidepressant effects that were sustained for up to a week after treatment (compared with a placebo) (Wilkinson et al. 2018). Other studies have shown ketamine can reduce suicidal ideation (Zanos et al. 2018).

Esketamine (Spravato, or S-ketamine) became the first drug approved by the FDA for treatment-resistant depression in 2019. Esketamine was also found to reduce suicidal ideation in depressed patients (Canuso et al. 2018). The FDA granted health-care providers the ability to prescribe Spravato for patients with suicidal ideation in 2019 as well.

# WHAT DOES LIFTING DEPRESSION LOOK LIKE?

Reddit user u/ocean6csgo described his experience with ketamine in the r/TherapeuticKetamine community:

> First. I'm really, really lucky. My depression and anxiety were gone almost immediately. I walked out saying, "Dang, I enjoyed that. I think I feel pretty damn good." And an hour later I was like, "I'm going to go eat healthy because I said I would in my trip session." Another hour later I put all my gro-

ceries away, and just ate a solidly healthy meal... Then I did all sorts of productive shit. Another hour later, I just wanted to call people and tell them how great I felt. While week one was the height of the height. I still feel great. I felt as if I didn't need to sweat the small stuff in life.

Life used to feel like pushing a rock uphill, and I thought that was normal. Turns out that's not normal, and life is a lot better than that.

My drive is back, and it just feels so nice to be in the driver's seat.

Emily Witt, author of the *New Yorker* piece, "Ketamine Is Going Mainstream: Are We Ready?" writes:

The next day, I felt different. I did some things I had put off for a long time, and stopped obsessing over other things that had monopolized my thoughts for weeks or months. Perhaps I had been primed to feel this way by the research I had read, but my state of mind seemed only indirectly related to anything I'd seen on my ketamine trip, and entirely unrelated to any kind of therapy. It seemed physical in nature. My mind was working the way I often wish it did. I had, in the past, tried to achieve this state of mind through drinking caffeine, through not drinking caffeine, through exercise, sleep, meditation, antidepressants, healthy eating, vitamin B12, magnesium, amphetamines, yoga. My mind had always seemed resistant to on-demand engineering. This new feeling was neither an afterglow nor a state of stimulation. It felt like stability. I didn't want to drink alcohol, or even coffee, out of a fear that the feeling would abandon me; I dreaded being thrown back into my ordinary mind. The feeling lasted a little more than two weeks, and then it went away. The memory of what it had felt like lingered a bit longer, and then it went away, too.

**THE KETAMINE HANDBOOK**

Witt also describes what this experience is like for others:

> He [Zachary] went home and did chores he had put off for years. "It was literally like entering life for the first time," he told me, comparing it to the process of color correction when making a film. "Ketamine color-corrected for my existence. I saw the world as it was, without this heavy gray mass."

Susan Gayhart described her experience for the *Boise Ketamine Clinic* blog:

> I was told I would probably know right away if the ketamine was going to work or not, and I did, within an hour. The anxiety I could never escape was lowered within an hour. I was alert and felt calm for the first time in my life. It was fast acting. My results were very obvious. Clearly I couldn't hide the fact that I felt better. You could hear it in my voice.

Another Reddit user, u/madscribbler, speaks to how ketamine helped him finally start living again:

> I've been on ketamine for 4.5 years. I have had 100 percent remission of rumination, depression, ideation, CPTSD, and almost all trigger situations nonstop. Ketamine has rebuilt my healthy synapses and relocated dendrites, so I'm able to cope with life in a healthy way and now view the world through an accurate lens showing love, support, compassion, and acceptance of me and who I am today.
>
> Ketamine improves cognition, memory, and mental flexibility, so damage caused by depression has been healed completely. This results in mental clarity, and an overall lighter feeling across life. Depression was a heavy blanket that weighed me down, unmotivated. Hard to start, harder to finish. Ketamine made my mind quieter; I no longer cycle on

unhealthy thoughts. I am no longer obsessed with suicide. I no longer ruminate.

I love life and live every minute. I feel joy and happiness now, and I'm very content the majority of the time. These past 4.5 years have been the best of my life.

## DEPRESSION & DOSING

The most commonly used subanesthetic antidepressant dose of ketamine is 0.5 mg per kilogram of body weight administered over a 40-minute infusion (Zarate et al. 2012).

Researchers note that smaller doses of ketamine may also act in a therapeutic manner. "There is some evidence for antidepressant responses achieved at doses as low as 0.1 mg/kg (5-minute IV infusion or intramuscular injection)...as reported in a small pilot double-blind, placebo-controlled crossover study in patients suffering from treatment-resistant depression" (Loo et al. 2016). Authors of the paper note that their findings "await replication in a larger study."

# ANTI-INFLAMMATORY

Ketamine can also exert anti-inflammatory effects. It does so by reducing the production of proinflammatory compounds called cytokines, thereby reducing inflammation.

Research has shown ketamine also decreases blood levels of interleukin 6 (IL-6), a cytokine produced in response to infections and tissue injury. High levels of IL-6 are associated with a number of conditions including poor postoperative surgical outcomes, inflammatory conditions such as arthritis, and, of course, depression (Zanos et al. 2018).

"That's good news for my patients with multiple sclerosis [MS] and other autoimmune diseases," says Adam Kaplin, a psychiatric consultant at Johns Hopkins's multiple sclerosis and transverse myelitis centers of excellence. Kaplin notes that 50 percent of patients with MS suffer from depression, adding that suicide is the third leading cause of death in patients with MS.

## ANTI-INFLAMMATORY DOSING

There is limited data on the use of ketamine for anti-inflammatory effects, but some studies suggest that low-dose ketamine may have potential as an anti-inflammatory agent.

In animal studies, subanesthetic doses of ketamine have been shown to reduce inflammation and oxidative stress in a variety of conditions, such as traumatic brain injury (Kopra at al. 2021).

A study of 20 healthy human volunteers found that a single dose of 0.5 mg/kg ketamine given intravenously produced a significant reduction in cytokine levels (Zanos et al. 2018).

More research is needed to determine the optimal dosing regimen for ketamine as an anti-inflammatory agent.

# KETAMINE DOSAGES AND METHODS OF ADMINISTRATION FOR CLINICAL USE AND SIDE EFFECTS IN HUMANS

| CLINICAL USES AND SIDE EFFECTS | ROUTE OF ADMINISTRATION | KETAMINE DOSE |
|---|---|---|
| General anesthesia | Intravenous | 1.0–2 mg/kg |
| | Intramuscular | 4–11 mg/kg |
| | Rectal | 8–10.6 mg/kg |
| | Oral | 500 mg (max)—sedation |
| | Intranasal | For esketamine: 3–9 mg/kg |
| Analgesia | Intravenous | 0.15 mg/kg |
| | Intramuscular | 0.5–1 mg/kg |
| | Intranasal | 2 x 10–50 mg |
| | Transdermal | 25 mg released throughout a 24-hour period |
| | Subcutaneous | 0.05–0.15 mg/kg per hour for 7 days |
| | Rectal | 10 mg/kg |
| | Oral | 2 mg/kg |
| | | 0.5 mg/kg |
| Anti-inflammation | Intravenous | 0.15–0.25 mg/kg |
| Antidepressant | Intravenous | 0.5 mg/kg; 40-min infusion |

CLINICAL EFFECTS

| CLINICAL USES AND SIDE EFFECTS | ROUTE OF ADMINISTRATION | KETAMINE DOSE |
|---|---|---|
| Dissociation | Intravenous | 0.3 mg/kg bolus* |
| Psychotomimetic effects in subjects with schizophrenia | Intravenous | 0.3 mg/kg bolus |
| | | 0.12 mg/kg bolus followed by a 60-min infusion of 0.65 mg/kg (total dose 0.77 mg/kg) |
| Cognitive and memory impairment | Intravenous | 40- to 120-min infusion of 0.4–0.8 mg/kg |
| | | 0.5 mg/kg bolus |
| | | infusion over length of testing (total dose variable) |
| Abuse (recreational use) | Intramuscular | 0.25–0.5 mg/kg bolus |
| | Intravenous | 1–2 mg/kg |
| | Intramuscular | 50–150 mg |
| | Oral | 100–500 mg |
| | Intranasal | 30–400 mg |

Source: Zanos et al. 2018

---

* A large, singular dose of a drug.

# Chapter 4

# INTRODUCING KETAMINE-ASSISTED PSYCHOTHERAPY (KAP)

This chapter will be devoted to learning all about ketamine-assisted psychotherapy (KAP) and how it works.

Ketamine was viewed as undesirable by many clinicians who believed its psychomimetic properties "limit clinical use" (Li and Vlisides 2016). The term "psychomimetic" describes drugs that mimic the effects of psychosis, a state in which subjects are not in touch with reality. Ketamine's psychomimetic properties are often compared to the effects of psychedelics and can include hallucinations, delusions, dissociative feelings, or strange somatic experiences.

A new school of thought, however, gradually emerged in contrast to the idea that the psychedelic aspects of the ketamine experience were undesirable. While some professionals argued ketamine's psychomimetic properties limited its use, others put forth the idea that these psychedelic effects made up a vital part of ketamine's therapeutic promise. In a 2019 research paper published in the *Journal of Psychoactive Drugs,* the authors of the paper opened with this assertion: "We believe ketamine can benefit patients with a wide variety of diagnoses when administered with psychotherapy and using its psychedelic properties without need for intravenous (IV) access" (Dore et al. 2019).

This belief has since been translated into a new practice known as ketamine-assisted psychotherapy (KAP).

KAP is a new mode of psychotherapy in which patients are administered ketamine and guided through a psychedelic experience with a licensed health-care professional in a supervised clinical setting. It's a combination of several kinds of therapy including cognitive behavioral therapy (CBT), psychodynamic therapy, and other self-improvement techniques. Psychodynamic therapy is your standard "talk" therapy. Cognitive behavioral therapy (CBT), on the other hand, is a specialized type of therapeutic approach that helps people identify and change maladaptive thoughts and behaviors. CBT is especially effective as it "promotes more balanced thinking to improve the ability to cope with stress" (Nakao et al. 2021). In fact, CBT is often thought of as the golden standard of psychological treatment (David et al. 2018).

KAP utilizes the introspective components of CBT and pairs them with ketamine's neuroplastic properties to help patients break free from trauma.

Researchers suggested that KAP is an effective method for treating patients suffering from depression, especially those with severe symptoms (Dore et al. 2019). Jennifer Dore et. al found that ketamine created enhanced benefits for patients that other antidepressants with no mind-altering effects did not provide (Dore et al. 2019). Parallels between ketamine and psilocybin, the psychoactive component of "magic mushrooms," led Dore's team to conclude mystical experiences were correlated with positive treatment outcomes, including improved mental health and overall well-being.

This reinforces the idea that the psychedelic experience itself is key to successful therapeutic outcomes.

Rather than search for a way to eliminate the psychedelic effects, KAP aims to utilize the psychedelic experience to help patients engage in introspective thought. The KAP experience posits the idea that subjects under the influence of ketamine may experience the absence of emotional constraints of the ordinary mind. The lack of these constraints helps patients achieve personal elucidation, or find deep meaning in their experiences. Anchoring, the process of gaining revelations and insights during the trip, can cause decreases in symptomatology for patients.

This idea of anchoring also supports the theory that ketamine can help induce neuroplasticity (Collo and Pich 2018).

"Ketamine has been shown to enhance neuroplasticity, which allows our mind to overcome rigid thinking and negative thought patterns," says Dr. Zand.

"By deconstructing rigid neurological and emotional barriers, psychedelic therapy promotes transformational shifts in perspective. Therapeutic exploration becomes easier and more efficient."

Let's dive into the concept of therapeutic exploration a little bit. How can we put a new spin on this age-old concept?

# ACCELERATED PSYCHOTHERAPY

According to Dr. Nazeer, a psychiatrist who founded the first psychiatric-led and psychiatric-based ketamine clinic in Chicago, if you have trauma in your past, that trauma might come back during an infusion of ketamine in vivid detail, but from a new perspective, and without all of the associated negative emotions that you have from that memory or trauma.

"That allows you to basically reframe the trauma and what it means to you," says Dr. Nazeer.

Dr. Nazeer also notes that this mode of therapy is akin to an "accelerated psychotherapy strategy," in which you can see yourself in a new light: "Sometimes people have what we call an ego death, which is kind of a rebirth. It's like the death of who you feel you are, your place in the world, and your ego…. And then it's like a rebirth of somebody in a new self-identification, and that's very powerful in psychotherapy." (For more on ego death, see page 44.)

# DRUG EFFICACY

KAP allows medical health-care professionals to address the *root* cause of the issues that cause depression, anxiety, and PTSD. This, in fact, represents a radical departure from the traditional model of treating depression. Rather than attempt to treat depression by correcting neurotransmitter levels, KAP and other psychedelic-assisted therapy modalities aim to induce changes in brain function that allow patients to have introspective, meaningful experiences with lasting positive outcomes. We can think of this concept expanding in terms of a shift from "drug efficacy" to "experience efficacy" (Schenberg 2018).

A number of studies have been conducted to assess the benefits associated with KAP. These studies include some which examined ketamine as a treatment for alcohol use disorder, gambling disorder, and even autism spectrum disorder.

# EXPLORING KETAMINE TREATMENT FOR ALCOHOL USE DISORDER

Alcohol use disorder is a chronic condition characterized by excessive drinking and difficulty controlling alcohol consumption. Ketamine is currently being studied as a potential treatment for this debilitating condition.

Krystal strikes again! The legendary ketamine researcher and his research team published an eight-week open-label pilot study investigating ketamine's antidepressant properties when administered with naltrexone, a medication for opioid use disorder, in 2019. Researchers put forth the idea that the antidepressant effects of ketamine might be dependent on opiate receptor stimulation. They concluded that a treatment which antagonized opiate receptors such as naltrexone combined with ketamine could be a viable strategy to "reduce addiction risk among patients with depression at risk for substance abuse." Their data even suggested the combination of the two drugs "might enhance the treatment of comorbid alcohol use disorder" (Krystal et al. 2019).

A 2020 pilot study published in the *American Journal of Psychiatry* sought to examine ketamine's effects on adults with alcohol dependence. Authors tested whether a lone administration of the drug—combined with motivational enhancement therapy—would affect drinking outcomes. Researchers discovered that a single infusion of ketamine was found to improve measures of drinking in persons concurrently enrolled in motivational enhancement therapy, "suggest[ing] new directions in integrated pharmacotherapy-behavioral treatments for alcohol use disorder" (Dakwar et. al 2019).

A randomized controlled trial assessing ketamine's impact on forty alcohol-dependent adults published in 2020 noted that subanesthetic doses of ketamine may be helpful for substance use disorders. Researchers found that ketamine administration led to "significant reduction" in at-risk drinking among subjects (Rothberg et al. 2020).

Further research is needed to replicate these promising results in larger samples.

# INVESTIGATING KETAMINE AS A THERAPEUTIC AID FOR GAMBLING DISORDER

Gambling disorder is often thought of as an impulse control disorder. Substance use disorders are also often thought of in this vein.

Interestingly enough, researchers have noted the two conditions share a number of similarities:

> Although distinct from one another, these disorders share similarities in phenomenology, etiology, pathophysiology, patient characteristics, and clinical outcomes. They can also be viewed as part of a continuum that spans from compulsivity to impulsivity, and they are characterized by harm avoidance as far as compulsion or risk-seeking for impulsivity. (Martinotti et al. 2021)

These conditions also share another trait: abnormalities in glutamate transmissions. Therefore, researchers have postulated the idea that ketamine, which can produce increases in glutamate, "could represent a valuable therapeutic option" (Martinotti et al. 2021).

A 2020 case study report following a 44-year-old man with a 20-year gambling addiction investigated ketamine's ability to impact his gambling habits. The subject underwent four sessions of IV ketamine at 0.5 mg/kg for two weeks. His gambling disorder symptoms dropped from a pretreatment PG-YBOCS score of 31 to a score of 7 after the second infusion (Grant and Chamberlain 2020). The Yale Brown Obsessive Compulsive Scale adapted for Pathological Gambling (PG-YBOCS) is a scoring a scoring system developed to measure the severity of pathological gambling symptoms.

## KETAMINE AND AUTISM SPECTRUM DISORDERS

Ketamine has been studied as a potential treatment for autism spectrum disorder (ASD), a neurodevelopmental disorder characterized by difficulties in social interaction, communication, and behavior.

A case study published in *The International Journal on Disability and Human Development* presented the tale of a patient with severe intellectual disabilities who experienced a "dramatic, albeit short-lived" remission of his symptoms following ketamine treatment (Kastner et al. 2016).

It is important to note that up to the date of publication, the studies investigating the use of ketamine as a treatment for ASD have been limited and inconclusive.

While the results so far have been promising, more research is needed to establish the long-term efficacy and safety of ketamine in the treatment of these conditions. Additional research is also needed to determine the optimal dose, frequency, and duration of ketamine treatment for each condition.

Despite ketamine's therapeutic promise, funding has been tragically limited. "Because the ketamine compound has been generic for decades, there isn't much funding supporting wide-scale clinical trials," says Dr. Zand.

## IS TELEHEALTH ESKETAMINE A GOOD THING?

Given the extensive list of concerns associated with Spravato, I cannot recommend patients opt for this form of ketamine.

I highly encourage anyone who's interested in therapeutic ketamine to seek out racemic ketamine whenever possible. Be sure to do your due diligence and ask your psychiatrist what kind of ketamine they can administer. Don't be afraid to call up plenty of psychiatrists, ketamine clinics, or health-care providers to get what you need, even if it takes a little more time. Find a compounding pharmacy that may be willing to help.

Access to ketamine via telehealth services is, in and of itself, a revolutionary new type of medicine that can quickly help many desperate patients in need. After all, some patients experience depression so debilitating that they are unable to leave the house. Other patients may not have health-care or cannot access it for a number of reasons as simple as lacking access to reliable transportation. And even if patients are lucky enough to have health care and access to transportation, many are ultimately at the mercy of health-care systems in which they may not receive access to care for weeks or months at a time.

Telehealth medicine removes these obstacles, reducing the amount of time someone has to wait before they can receive access to care. This aspect of it is very much a good thing. However, this system is also rife with the potential for abuse. It still remains to be seen whether or not Spravato is a good alternative for patients experiencing depression in the long run. Patients at home can also easily lie about the severity of symptoms in order to access dosages that go far beyond therapeutic value, leading to potential substance abuse.

Although there are some very real concerns in place regarding telehealth implementation, it is undeniable that telehealth medicine represents an important shift in psychiatry, giving access to patients who may not normally have any. The advent of ketamine telehealth therapy in this manner has likely saved more lives than we can count.

When the pandemic hit and my depression intensified, ketamine—in its racemic form—saved my life. It somehow reduced the terror I felt at the prospect of leaving the house or interacting with people, allowing me to leave the house without fear for the first time in years.

I can't imagine where I would be today without ketamine, and I'm sure many others out there feel the same. But would Spravato have had comparable effects? Something in me seriously doubts it.

Careful, well-thought-out policies must be put in place soon to ensure that the field of telehealth medicine remains a safe, viable alternative for patients who struggle to get access to care. (For more on the ethical concerns of telehealth services, see page 109.)

# KAP IN REAL LIFE

What does KAP look like in real life? KAP can be broken down into three different stages: preparation, treatment, and integration.

## STAGE 1: PREPARATION SESSION

The first part of KAP therapy is centered around preparing the patient for the experience. This starts off with a discussion between a patient and a psychotherapist or facilitator. What is the patient's reason for coming in? What issues are they intending to address? This is when a patient might discuss their trauma and relationship history, and when the facilitator would conduct and review a general psychological assessment. Contraindications, or conditions not suitable for ketamine treatment, are addressed at this time. It's also imperative that a sense of trust, or rapport, is established between the facilitator and the patient, according to Dr. Nazeer.

"You don't want to just go into it with somebody you don't know," Dr. Nazeer warns. "If something comes up and you don't have that trust, you don't feel that rapport with them, that kind of impacts psychological safety and it can be a worse outcome."

Facilitators do their best to try and give patients an idea of what to expect during their psychedelic experience with respect to dissociation. If you recall from page 29, dissociation is when subjects can feel disconnected from their bodies or surroundings. This is often described by patients as a dream-like or trance state that can be accompanied by a sense of euphoria. As activity in the DMN is reduced, patients can begin to feel more connected to their environment.

While many patients come into the therapy with an understanding of ketamine's mind-altering effects, it's important for the facilitator to prepare them as much as possible for such an unusual experience.

Evgeny Krupitsky (MD, PhD), a vice director for research and a chief of the Department of Addictions at V.M. Bekhterev National Medical Research Center of Psychiatry and Neurology in St. Petersburg, describes this process:

> We tell the patient that they will enter some unusual states of consciousness and that they may feel detached from their

body....We also instruct them to surrender fully to the experience.

Moreover, we attempt to explain to the patients that the psychedelic session may induce important insights concerning the resolution of their problems and the reorientation of their system of values, their notions of self, and the world around them, and the meaning of their life.

Discussing therapeutic goals ahead of sessions with your mental health-care provider is another important part of the preparation process. Adam Mitchell describes this process in detail:

During the preparation phase, the alliance between patient-participant and therapist-facilitator begins: a patient's reason for coming in to participate with the treatment is explored. Trauma history, psychological and relational factors affecting the participant are reviewed and understood by the facilitator, as well as what efforts had been taken in the past and their limits are shared by the participant to their facilitator.

Notice how Mitchell uses terms like "alliance." In addition to outlining therapeutic goals, it's of vital importance for health-care professionals to establish a sense of trust and rapport with their patients before administration.

# STAGE 2: THE TRIP ITSELF

The second stage of KAP is the administration of the ketamine itself under controlled medical supervision in a safe, friendly environment. This can take place in a number of different settings ranging from a physician's private office to one of the many ketamine clinics sprouting up across the country. Stage 2 is conducted by two physicians, a psychotherapist and an anesthesiologist, because some complications and side effects such as increased blood pressure are possible.

The dose and form of ketamine administered can have profound impacts on the nature of treatment.

"For some people the form of ketamine matters a lot," says Dr. Nazeer.

Dr. Nazeer points out that IM ketamine can feel more intense and dissociative. As such it has a sudden drop off, or wearing-off period. Intravenous (IV) ketamine, on the other hand, is "a little smoother," with a more gradual comedown. Which experience is "best" comes down to a matter of personal preference.

## IM VS IV

As mentioned previously, IM is the administration of ketamine via intramuscular injection. IV, or intravenous ketamine, has a higher bioavailability, though IM can be more intense and dissociative.

Ketamine behaves differently at different doses. At low doses, ketamine is "more meditative and empathogenic," says Dr. Zand. At more moderate doses, it "can start to provide perspective shifts through altered states of consciousness." Even higher doses can result in "a psychedelic experience with potentially profound benefits for subconscious awareness and ego-actualization."

In other words, it's a choose-your-own-adventure game. Choose a low dose and you'll feel a sensation akin to being stoned: an easygoing, relaxed euphoria. Increase your dosage to gain access to profound, psychedelic-like states for mind-bending epiphanies.

"Our clinic prefers intramuscular injections over IV administrations of ketamine, due to the longer and more substantial experiential effect of IM over IV treatments," says Adam Mitchell, Director of

Clinical Research at My Self Wellness (https://myselfwellness. center), a ketamine therapy treatment center based in Florida.

Mitchell goes on to explain that IV drips slowly elevate blood serum levels of ketamine. Intramuscular administration, however, is optimally performed using two shots, the second of which is administered approximately 10 to 25 minutes after the first. These IM shots get blood serum levels to higher levels more swiftly than IV, says Mitchell. The second shot, too, is key in the therapeutic experience for patients as it keeps the "therapeutic window" of patient experience open longer than an equivalent amount of ketamine administered via IV.

"The IM shot immerses our patients into the 'depth' of the experience more quickly than IV," Mitchell explains:

> Our clinic notes the therapeutic insights our patients draw from the experience they have during their sessions. We aim to give our patients a deep journey, longer than IV patients may access, and to help them take time to integrate. With these factors, our clinic accommodates patients for longer than many IV clinics do.

In other words, Mitchell's clinic opts for IM shots as they keep the therapeutic window, or mindset in which patients may be in a neuroplastic state, open for longer. This allows subjects to spend as much time as possible in this introspective state, which can help them create new neural pathways.

While Mitchell's practice is based on extensive patient experience, he reminds us that ketamine therapy is still being investigated for best practices. Mitchell is careful to routinely follow up with patients to be sure his clinic is incorporating the best clinical practices possible. Patients at MY Self Wellness also have the option of choosing IV treatment if they prefer.

Once patients are adequately prepared, administration sessions can begin. Set and setting are two vital components for successful administration. These terms refer to the environment in which administration will occur (setting) as well as the patient's prospective outlook on their therapeutic goals (set). Do they feel comfortable? Safe? The importance of setting is emphasized by creating a peaceful setting for patients. Many of the rooms KAP is conducted in typically share features, such as comfortable furniture, including zero gravity chairs and lots of pillows and blankets to create the warmest, most comfortable setting possible. Patients are often given eye masks to wear and meditative music is played. Music is said to enhance the ketamine experience.

In-office health-care professionals at ketamine clinics typically include a psychiatrist to monitor reactions as well as an anesthesiologist to monitor vitals. As a patient enters their first session, they are typically supervised by a trained clinical professional who is present not only to monitor the patient's vitals or assist in any cases of unexpected reactions, but to provide support and comfort, often taking notes to better help the patient eventually make sense of their journey.

One doctor running a ketamine therapy clinic out of Los Angeles reassures his patients: "If you ever feel like you want some grounding, you can put your hand out to your side like this"—he demonstrated—"or on your shoulder, and I'll come touch your hand or shoulder for a moment" (Krekow 2022). Patients often report that these health-care professionals play a huge role in helping them manage pretreatment jitters. I know this because I was terrified my first time, but once my physician sat next to me and smiled patiently, I knew I'd be okay.

Patients can experience a wide range of responses during treatment, ranging from a state of peaceful meditation to a full-on psychedelic, ego-dissolving trip. Psychotherapists or facilitators remain on hand or nearby to assist patients with anything that may come up during their experience. Headphones and eye masks are often given to patients to help them focus and relax.

One of the most common universal experiences patients go through in ketamine clinics is a resistance to the journey. This can manifest in the form of feeling overwhelmed by visual or sensory elements like hallucinations, or as outright panic. It can also manifest as a desire to run away from any deep-seated problems that may bubble to the forefront of the mind at this time.

Regardless of the type of discomfort a patient faces, health-care professionals (and experienced ketamine users alike) often encourage patients to surrender to the experience. Surrender in this sense can be thought of as accepting whatever is happening, whether it's good or bad, allowing whatever sensations or images that come up to wash over you.

Sessions typically last 45 minutes to an hour. The intensity of the trip, or the psychedelic aspects of the experience, varies wildly depending on the unique body composition of the individual. I myself have an extremely low tolerance to ketamine and have felt therapeutic effects from as little as sublingual doses of 25 mg. Other patients report needing doses as high as 400 mg to feel equivalent effects.

The trip itself is different for everyone. Many people often report feeling a gentle euphoria as they may begin to notice changes in their visual field. Colors may appear to be brighter, or subjects may register new types of movements in their surroundings. Patients may experience auditory or visual hallucinations. A physical sense of lightness often described as "floaty" can produce the strange feeling that your body is floating or weightless. I feel my analytical, ruminative mind slip away and become hushed, quiet, at peace.

"My sense of my human life and body was dialed down to almost zero," writes Reddit user u/0ldboy67. He elaborates on the nature of his trip in a post on r/TherapeuticKetamine:

> I was in different realities, and my "normal" life was scarcely even dim memory—like a prior, irrelevant lifetime thousands of years ago which I could recall if I wanted to (but didn't want to). It felt like it would go on forever, and when the time came to leave that realm I didn't want to....
>
> As I reintegrated into my daily life, it's in a different perspective than before the ketamine. It's as if dimensions of being of which I hadn't been aware were opened to me and integrated into myself, filling in cracks and healing broken places.

Another user in the therapeutic ketamine subreddit, u/EER_ESQ, describes his first ketamine journey in more colorful terms:

> The trip was dreamlike, but not dreamlike. Dreams have a "reality" to them—i.e. my dreams have people, places, things. The ketamine trip did not. Instead, I saw colors and shapes and patterns. The colors and patterns would shift and move. I felt as if I was a part of the color and pattern. My body felt like it was moving along with whatever was going on around me. Sometimes spinning, sometimes being pulled along a current, sometimes floating. It was unlike anything I've ever experienced. I also felt very "light" during the experience and had a sense of wonder through it all.

Patients slowly "come back" from their experiences, a recovery period which can take one to two hours. Grogginess is a common side effect as the effects of the drug wear off. Subjects can feel tired or dreamy. They also may experience cloudy thinking, nausea, disorientation, or even a feeling of drunkenness.

Reddit user u/manwithninebuttocks paints a picture:

Towards the *very* end of the drip I started to gain some sense of reality and could wiggle my fingers and toes. A minute later the nurse was taking off my IV and reality was fully there. Super quick.

Redditor u/EER_ESQ writes:

After coming to, I felt pretty disoriented. It was like being drunk. I felt the spins and could not stand or walk. I sat on a chair in the room for at least 15 minutes before I was OK enough to walk out to the waiting room. I sat in the waiting room for probably another 30 minutes. After that, I felt fine to walk out of the building. I still felt foggy and a bit in a daze, but I was able to speak to my wife normally and was fine eating lunch on the way home.

Once subjects are more lucid, however, they're often in an introspective mood—excited by the new insights they've gained and eager to share their experience.

This is when patients will typically begin relaying their experience to the facilitator. Some facilities will have creative tools such as journals and markers available for this purpose. Patients may also be asked to write a detailed report describing their journey. These types of activities help patients integrate their experiences into their everyday lives.

# STAGE 3: INTEGRATION

The therapeutic effects of ketamine aren't solely due to the psychedelic experience. Integration, a form of psychotherapy in which facilitators help patients integrate any insights they've gained during their trips, is absolutely imperative to ketamine's therapeutic success. Mitchell paints a picture of what the integration process looks like at My Self Wellness:

> After each medication session, a facilitator helps patient integrate their experience and adjust to the external world. Prior to each subsequent session, the facilitator reviews how the participant has been since their last session, challenges and insights it may have brought up.

My Self Wellness also provides participants with the option to engage in integration-focused support groups following treatment.

Integration can pose a challenge for patients, especially those with more chronic or long-term treatment-resistant conditions. Dr. Nazeer illustrates the manner in which this challenge presents itself to patients and their families:

> Some people, let's say they're depressed for 20 years, they've tried every treatment and nothing's improved…suddenly they're getting a new approach about how they think about themselves and their life and it's healthier and they're not sick anymore. That's a big adjustment for the family, the caregivers, the spouse's loved ones, and for the patients themselves. How do they reframe their identity? What do you do with your newfound neuroplastic state and healthy kind of mental health? What do you do with that? How do you integrate that into your life?

Mitchell also stresses the importance of doing the work yourself following treatment.

"Although ketamine treatment 'works like magic' for some, it is not a silver bullet for all conditions," Mitchell says. "Miraculous as ketamine may be, the work YOU do is imperative," he continues.

# MAINTENANCE & DOSING

While more research is ultimately needed here, current KAP models typically recommend a treatment course of six to eight treatments over the course of three to four weeks. Patients can then experience a reduction of pain. According to Mitchell, this includes physical, mental, and emotional pain, diminished to a degree where they find future treatments completely unnecessary.

Mitchell says some patients will soon find that their reliance on psychiatric and pain medication or chemical abuse behaviors has "disappeared entirely." Other patients may benefit from a set of "booster" treatments administered a few months later. This is what's known as a maintenance schedule.

"It remains to be determined if two to three treatment cycles a year may be more effective and longer lasting than singular treatment cycles," continues Mitchell.

Some providers are now allowing patients to take home ketamine, generally in the form of oral tablets. This practice, however, is not without its own concerns.

"While I do believe that take-home ketamine can be managed appropriately in certain instances, I do have concerns about any home dosing that is lacking in professional support and follow-up," says Robison. "There's an adage among mental health practitioners that you've got to feel it to heal it. And the reality is, sometimes you feel worse before you feel better. For this reason, I won't even consider take-home dosing unless we've done work with the client in the office first."

# ADDRESSING KETAMINE AND KAP MISCONCEPTIONS

Rife with therapeutic promise though it may be, KAP treatment is subject to critics who cite fear of misuse.

Dr. Nazeer also added that he had not seen a single instance of ketamine misuse over five or six years and 5,000 treatments utilizing ketamine.

"We are doing it in a controlled environment. We are not sending ketamine home with patients, which I think can be problematic if you don't have mental health oversight, psychiatric involvement, or mental health specialists involved," he adds.

Mitchell concurs, noting that while some patients may believe ketamine can be used recreationally in therapeutic ways, "personal, unsupervised use of 'street' ketamine (no matter the purity) is not the same as its therapeutic applications. Increased risk makes it challenging for sufferers to self-treat with ketamine outside of a therapeutic framework."

The list of potential risks is long, but it includes the following:

○ Dangers of contraindications: a patient may have a condition, such as high blood pressure, which makes them a bad candidate for ketamine. In said case, ketamine administration could prove to be dangerous. We'll cover this more in a bit.

○ Risk of developing psychological or physiological addiction.

○ Lack of education about dosing. Ketamine's effects are notoriously dose-dependent and vary depending on the unique body chemistry of every individual. One person's "just right" dose may prove to be unbearable for another. Dosing recreational ketamine is extremely challenging and almost impossible to do with accuracy.

Many of the horror stories I heard about ketamine were based on the fear of entering a "K-hole," a dissociated state so deep users would appear to be completely unresponsive. This is, of course, in line with what research tells us: that larger doses of ketamine produce a sedating effect. Subanaesthetic doses (less than surgical doses) offer the best therapeutic outcomes, and will not generally produce a "K-hole" state.

# CONCERN AND CONTRAINDICATIONS

Like any other modality, KAP treatment comes with its own unique set of concerns. Therefore, patients should carefully review their medical histories with providers to ensure they are good candidates for treatment. It is essential to do so to avoid contraindications, or conditions that suggest candidates may not be suitable for a particular kind of treatment.

Mitchell cites the following conditions as those which are currently contraindicated for ketamine use/treatment. These include:

- significant physiological dysfunction of heart, lungs, spinal fluid, liver, or kidney functioning
- high blood pressure and intraocular pressure
- active psychosis, delirium, or intoxication
- active or past ketamine abuse

## PSYCHOSIS AND MANIA

A family history of psychosis or substance abuse may deter some providers from greenlighting ketamine treatment.

As a general guideline, people with cognitive and emotional conditions associated with disorganized or diminished ego strength (such as psychosis or mania) are not good candidates for psychedelics, according to Dr. Robison.

"At Numinus, we do a thorough medical and psychiatric screening," says Dr. Robison.

However, patients evaluated by medical professionals with certain aforementioned conditions may still be able to undergo KAP.

Dr. Zand has noted that he has successfully treated a schizophrenic patient (a condition characterized by psychosis) with low-dose ketamine. He has also used ketamine clinically for many patients previously diagnosed with bipolar disorder.

"For those with severe mania or a history of psychosis, it is important to avoid higher doses of ketamine which can induce further mania or psychosis," adds Dr. Zand. "In this population, we are more focused on the meditative quality of lower doses."

Can ketamine itself trigger psychosis?

"While the nature of ketamine on development trajectories of psychiatric risk is not yet known, more research is needed," says Mitchell. "At present, it does not seem as though ketamine poses the same risk of triggering psychopathology which psychedelics like LSD, psilocybin and others have."

Everyone's somatic responses, however, will differ, which is why you should always consult with a medical health professional before trying out ketamine.

In my experience there is no one-size fits all criteria that says "having X condition is always bad for ketamine treatment." I've known people with no mental or physical health conditions become terribly addicted to ketamine. I've also seen dope addicts that would sell their grandmama's teeth for a hit pass up ketamine in favor of other drugs. I've known patients with BPD use ketamine with total success. Hell, Dr. Zand's even treated schizophrenic patients with ketamine before, so we can't rule out psychosis completely and totally, can we?

There are no rules...yet.

# INTERACTION WITH OTHER COMMON DRUGS

Another potential area of concern involves ketamine's interactions with other common drugs.

Ketamine is metabolized by cytochrome P450 (CYP) enzymes. These enzymes metabolize many conventional drugs such as diazepam (Valium), tricyclic antidepressants such as amitriptyline (Elavil), and antihistamines including terfenadine (Bibi 2008).

Therefore, any drugs consumed that induce or inhibit these enzymes will affect exposure to ketamine. Grapefruit juice is one known culprit. It inhibits CYP enzymes, increasing the bioavailability of drugs, which can produce serious adverse reactions.

The lesson? ALWAYS consult with a medical health professional before dabbling with drugs.

# SIDE EFFECTS

Long-term misuse of ketamine can result in a number of adverse side effects. These include the following:

- psychological dependence or abuse
- cognitive difficulties such as brain atrophy and encephalopathy (Liu et al. 2021)
- liver-gallbladder symptoms, such as abnormal liver function
- urinary symptoms such as increased frequency of urination
- hydronephrosis, or the swelling of kidneys, due to a buildup of urine
- chronic kidney injury
- renal failure (Liu et al. 2021)
- changes in brain anatomy, including reduced gray matter volume and less white matter integrity
- decreased connectivity between the thalamocortical and corticocortical regions of the brain, which "may explain some of its [ketamine's] long-term cognitive and psychiatric side effects, such as memory impairment and executive functioning" (Strous et al. 2022)

# Chapter 5

# ACCESSING KETAMINE THERAPY

Since the early 2000s, there's been a huge proliferation of ketamine treatment options available to those in need. And while this may seem to be a good thing, there are definitely a few areas of concern to address. Not all providers are created equal.

"If you are not screened well—and ketamine's not for everybody—it can open up other symptoms and it can make you feel worse and unsupported after," says Dr. Nazeer.

Screening, however, is only one vital part of the process. Here are a few best practices to help you find the right provider for you.

## DO YOUR HOMEWORK

While Johnson & Johnson has a nifty Spravato provider finder tool online, there aren't many other tools you can use to search for and compare ketamine providers. That means the onus of doing the research is in your hands.

"Consult research reviews and look for local clinics which provide ketamine treatments AND are well reviewed/regarded," says Dr. Nazeer, who has overseen almost 5,000 ketamine treatments.

You should also give some thought to researching the different forms of ketamine and assessing which may be best for you. Does the idea of a more intense trip appeal to you? Intravenous or intramuscular may be your best bet. Or are you keen on the lowest dose possible? Oral dosing may be a better fit. Consider all of your options carefully. You should also know the average out-of-pocket cost for six to eight ketamine sessions (the recommended course of treatment) generally ranges from $5,000 to $10,000.

Not sure where to start? You can find a map detailing locations of ketamine clinics around the country and a map of compounding pharmacies offering custom ketamine formulations at https://ketamineclinicsdirectory.com.

# WORK WITH YOUR INSURANCE

I know what you're thinking: can insurance even cover ketamine treatment? The answer is a little complicated.

Some insurers may cover ketamine treatment in strange ways. Certain providers, for instance, may only cover the initial psychiatric assessment you go in for to determine if ketamine treatment is right for you. Others may cover the cost of FDA-approved options such as Spravato, but only after a *significant* amount of legwork.

Your best bet in this journey is to try and find ways your insurance company can help cover the cost of treatment. And since there's no place that currently lists which providers cover which aspects of treatment, the only way to find out that information is to contact providers yourself directly. In my case, I had to contact my mental health provider, Optum, rather than my direct health-care provider, Oscar. I called Optum and told them I was interested in receiving ketamine treatment and therapy. I asked them to explain to me what I had to do to be eligible for treatment, what expenses might be covered, and what providers I could find in my area. They then connected me with Mindful Health Solutions, a health-care provider specializing in treating depression with innovative options, including TMS, esketamine, and ECT. Transcranial magnetic stimulation (TMS) is a type of noninvasive procedure that uses magnetic fields to stimulate nerve cells for patients with treatment-resistant depression. Electroconvulsive therapy (ECT) refers to a psychiatric treatment that uses electricity to treat certain mental health conditions.

There are, however, many hurdles to overcome here. I had to provide evidence to my insurance company that I had tried (and been failed by) several different antidepressants before I could be approved for coverage. Even after doing so, I was then asked to provide proof that I had been in therapy for the last five years. And since Spravato is the only form of ketamine that's currently FDA approved for depression, it can only be accessed by, well, patients who have pretty severe treatment-resistant depression. You may encounter the same when seeking treatment and be asked to prove you have unsuccessfully tried several antidepressants before you can be eligible for Spravato.

One viable option that worked very well for me was to have insurance cover a portion of treatment—the initial psychiatric evaluation. I was told IV or intramuscular ketamine treatments would not be covered by insurance. Spravato was an option…but I wasn't especially keen to try it.

The psychiatrist I saw who was willing to prescribe ketamine was able to find a compounding pharmacist in the area who created ketamine oral tablets for me to take home. Insurance didn't cover it all—I did have to pay out of pocket for the tablets—but since ketamine had been around for so long, the cost was only $50 a month for a daily 25 mg prescription. You may be able to work out an arrangement like this by talking to your health-care provider, generally a psychiatrist. You may also find some providers are skittish about prescribing ketamine and may be more hesitant to do so. My advice? Keep looking for providers until you find someone who is willing to help.

And of course, your mileage may vary wildly depending on your state, insurance plan, and unique needs. I was able to receive ketamine therapy in the state of Oregon after having proved I had unsuccessfully tried several antidepressants. Treatment was in the form of oral troches (lozenges) that I took home and administered daily, with a health-care provider monitoring my first administration session in-office.

That doesn't seem to be the case, however, in the state of California. Despite already proving I had unsuccessfully tried a litany of different antidepressants, at the time of writing this, my insurance company claims that I have to *currently* be on an antidepressant in order to qualify for Spravato treatment.

Needless to say, since the data on Spravato is misleading and the effects of antidepressants can be so severe, I did not opt for this route moving forward.

# POTENTIAL RED FLAGS

Dr. Nazeer has provided us with a few indicators that prospective ketamine patients should keep an eye out for.

The bare minimum standard for ketamine therapy "should include some sort of psychotherapist involvement even if there's not a medical psychiatric presence there," says Dr. Nazeer. He adds that treatment should also include somebody who is able to prepare you, give you integration therapy, and monitor you afterward.

"A lot of clinics might just be cash only, no mental health involvement, and no follow-up or no other services they can add to it, no proper integration. Those are all three red flags," he warns.

Another red flag is if the provider says that "they have a special blend or formulation in their ketamine—especially if it's considered secret or proprietary—and are adding it to your ketamine treatment, not telling you what it is," says Dr. Nazeer. "That's a huge red flag that goes against all the established published guidelines from American Society of Ketamine Physicians and APA, that it should be sticking to where the evidence is."

Dr. Nazeer is also wary of telehealth ketamine treatment in which providers send you ketamine to be used at home.

"If somebody prescribes you three to five days of ongoing home ketamine after you do your initial treatments in the clinic and there's no real follow-up, they give you a larger supply of home ketamine— that is also a red flag because there is no data to support its use and maintenance for depression, PTSD, or any mental health condition when taking ketamine regularly," Dr. Nazeer continues. "I believe that doing it in the clinic and keeping the goal to have the least amount possible, the most comprehensive support structure, and leveraging your insurance as well is the best option."

Since therapeutic ketamine is still so new, best practices are still currently being evaluated. Whether or not ketamine is best if taken at home still has to be determined; however, a 2022 research paper found at-home, sublingual ketamine telehealth to be "a safe and effective treatment for moderate to severe anxiety and depression" (Hull et al. 2022).

# CURRENT KETAMINE PROVIDERS

As of December 2022, these are the most well-known ketamine providers in the United States. I've also included brief notes summarizing what I know and have heard through word of mouth about each provider.

## SMITH KETAMINE SERVICES

**Type of ketamine offered:** Racemic ketamine sublingual troche (oral tablet). Other routes may be available in the future.

Head to the r/TherapeuticKetamine subreddit and it won't take long before you hear praise for Dr. Smith. Smith Ketamine Services (smithfamilymd.com) is one of the first private providers I have come across that is known for helping patients access ketamine treatment. They're also one of the most affordable options out there, with treatment options available for as low as $250 a month. Smith Ketamine Services are telehealth, meaning you'll be evaluated by an MD and given medication to take within the comfort of your own home. Prescriptions for ketamine issued by Smith Ketamine Services are sent off to compounding pharmacies near your location; patients pay for their ketamine supply at the pharmacy.

## JOYOUS

**Type of ketamine offered:** Racemic ketamine buccal troche (an oral tablet meant to be dissolved in your cheek).

One of the newest names in the ketamine industry, Joyous (www.joyous.team) is attempting to make a name for itself by offering radically affordable ketamine treatment. And unlike many of its contemporaries, Joyous focuses on delivering low-dose ketamine to patients. Treatment plans include an assessment, telehealth consultation, medication delivery, access to the Joyous Care team, and tools for $129 a month with no commitment necessary. Joyous also notes that they "accept HSA and FSA funds if you utilize those accounts in your health care."

So what's dosing like with Joyous? It's determined by artificial intelligence, apparently. In order to learn more about their program, I spoke with Joyous a few days ago as a prospective patient. Lexus Rogers, my nurse practitioner, explained over Zoom that Joyous's dosing protocol was AI driven. Joyous collects data from the patients in a number of ways, utilizing everything from a long initial patient questionnaire I filled out online to sending out daily texts asking patients about their mood levels. This data, especially the daily texts, Rogers explained, would then be input into Joyous's AI system. The Joyous AI then suggests the optimal dose for each patient depending on their unique needs.

# BETTER U CLINIC

**Type of ketamine offered:** Racemic oral ketamine. Esketamine Spravato available in-person in select states.

Founded by Dr. Zand, the Better U Clinic (www.betterucare.com) is another telehealth ketamine program available for at-home care. Head to their site to complete an online assessment. You'll then be scheduled for an appointment with a clinician who will craft your treatment plan and answer any questions you may have. The Better U program offers "therapeutic guidance, safety protocols, breathwork, virtual treatment preparation, and one-on-one integration coaching" for patients to get the most out of sessions. Two different plans are available: the "Introduction" plan (4 sessions for $596) or the "Transformation" plan (8 sessions for $1032). Financing options are also available on the site.

Better U is available in the following states: Nevada, California, Florida, Colorado, Arizona, Washington, and Texas. It's also available in Utah and Idaho, but these states will require an initial in-office visit.

# FIELD TRIP HEALTH

**Type of ketamine offered:** Racemic ketamine sublingual lozenges (Canada) or IM (United States).

Field Trip Health (www.fieldtriphealth.com) is a health and wellness company that offers guests the ability to experience a ketamine trip in the comfort of their clinics. Clinics here are specially designed to reduce feelings of discomfort or anxiety, and are equipped with a number of features including noise-canceling headphones, specially curated playlists, and weighted blankets. Their in-person ketamine assisted psychotherapy program includes preparation, exploratory sessions when ketamine is administered, and integration sessions. You can find their clinics in a number of different cities across the US and Canada, including:

- Chicago
- Fredericton
- Los Angeles
- New York
- San Diego
- Seattle
- Toronto
- Vancouver
- Washington, DC

While the Field Trip Health model is very appealing, the cost is sky high. Three different levels of service are available: Individual, Individual + Extra Support, and Support Plus. Each plan includes 13 sessions. Individual plans are cited as costing $5,250, with $6,750 for the Individual + Extra Support tier and $7,250 for the Support Plus option. Even more suspect is the asterisk on the payment plan section that says, "*Prices shown are based on 0% APR at 24 months. Rates are based on credit and subject to an eligibility

check. Down payment may be required. In the US, visit hellowalnut
.com/apply to view financing options."

## MY KETAMINE HOME (POWERED BY NUE LIFE)

**Type of ketamine offered:** Racemic ketamine oral sublingual
tablet.

Another ketamine telehealth provider is My Ketamine Home. My
Ketamine Home provides patients with oral ketamine tablets they
can take at home. They offer free initial consultations to help you
determine if their program is a good fit at myketaminehome.com/
get-started. I like the fact that they are transparent about dosing on
the site. Doses are determined by their medical team based on real
patient data and your personal health conditions. These typically
range from 2 to 7 milligrams per kilogram of body weight (mg/kg).

Several different treatment options are available. Their option that
best resembles traditional ketamine protocols consists of six treatments over several weeks. Called the Stabilize program, this will set
you back $1,399. The next service tier, the Complete program, con-
sists of the initial six Stabilize experiences followed by three months
of maintenance, providing a single shipment of twelve doses to be
spread across three months for $2,999.

## NUMINUS

**Type of ketamine offered:** Racemic ketamine oral rapid dissolving
tablet for initial doses, nasal spray for supplemental doses. Also
offers IM and esketamine (Spravato).

Dr. Reid Robison is the chief clinical officer at Numinus (numinus.
com), a mental health-care company specializing in psychedelic-assisted therapy and research. With locations in Vancouver,
Montreal, Toronto, Arizona, and Utah, Numinus offers a number of

different services, including ketamine therapy. Treatment options are flexible, with patients being able to opt for experiences that include a guiding therapist or self-guided sessions. You can learn more about Numinus's care team on their site. Interested patients can get started by booking an initial consultation call.

## MY SELF WELLNESS (AVAILABLE ONLY IN SOUTHWEST FLORIDA)

**Type of ketamine offered: Racemic ketamine IV and IM. Nasal spray offered in conjunction with psychiatry.**

My Self Wellness (myselfwellness.center) is a ketamine-assisted therapy provider that operates in Florida. Treatment is not covered by insurance; however, financing options are available, with treatments starting at $69/month.

## MINDBLOOM

**Type of ketamine offered:** Racemic ketamine sublingual tablet.

Although Mindbloom was one of the first companies to launch in this space, its reputation is less than stellar. I've seen many, many people complain about their experiences with Mindbloom, citing a lack of customer service and high prices.

Mindbloom offers six (oral, also called sublingual) ketamine treatments, a "Bloombox" (containing items including a blood pressure cuff, eye mask, and journal), two clinician consults, three guided sessions with unlimited messaging, and unlimited group integration sessions "from $89 a week billed monthly for three months." The exact cost of treatment is not apparent when viewing the site: $89/week per month, or $1,068 for three months. Scroll down to the bottom of the pricing page, however, and you'll see a chart that lists Mindbloom treatment as $1,158. Curiously enough, insurance reimbursements are listed as one of the Mindbloom program's benefits, though you'll find a convenient little asterisk there denoting "subject to insurance provider's approval" at the bottom of the page. Mindbloom also cites that HSA/FSA savings are available, again with an asterisk denoting this is ultimately "subject to card issuer's approval."

Mindbloom also offers an add-on option for those who are interested in 1:1 virtual integration coaching, with one 45-minute session costing an additional $59.

I could not find anything regarding dosing on Mindbloom's site.

## JOHNSON & JOHNSON: SPRAVATO

**Type of ketamine offered:** Esketemine

This one is a bit tricky; after all, research tentatively suggests racemic ketamine, rather than its lone S-enantiomer, is best suited for treating depression. But if you're desperate for treatment and are looking for a ketamine treatment option insurance may cover, you may want to consider Spravato. Johnson & Johnson has a handy map you can use to find a Spravato treatment center near you that you can access at www.spravato.com/find-a-center.

## TRIPSITTER.CLINIC

**Type of ketamine offered:** Racemic ketamine oral rapid dissolving tablet and intranasal spray.

This is another ketamine telehealth service that offers patients a tablet or nasal spray version of ketamine. For $599/month, their Ketamine-Enhanced Therapy Access program includes the following:

○ A medical evaluation with your prescribing physician

- Prescribed medication shipped to your door
- A pre-medication preparation session with a trained specialist
- Connection with a Tripsitter for treatment sessions
- Integration sessions to support you between doses—either one-on-one or in groups—with your Tripsitter

# NUE.LIFE

**Type of ketamine offered:** Racemic ketamine oral sublingual formation.

Nue.life's approach combines ketamine therapy, an interactive companion app, and virtual aftercare programs to help patients in need. They also offer several program tiers, including the "Nue. reset" 1-month subscription (six ketamine experiences, four group integration sessions, and one "health coaching session") for $1,399, as well as a "Nue.you" four-month subscription (18 ketamine experiences, 16 group integration sessions, and 4 health coaching sessions) for $2,999.

# KETAMD (ONLY AVAILABLE IN FLORIDA)

**Type of ketamine offered:** Racemic ketamine oral tablet.

KetaMD is a telehealth medicine platform that provides ketamine treatments administered at home. Head to their treatments tab and you'll spy a video of celebrity fan Lamar Odum. A former pro basketball player, Odum has publicly spoken about using ketamine treatment to help him with addiction.

KetaMD treatment packages include the following:

- KetaMD companion app
- KetaMD welcome kit
- Medical consultation
- Shipped medication
- Dedicated care concierge
- Treatment preparation

- KetaMD eye mask and blood pressure monitor
- Virtual ketamine treatments monitored by KetaMD certified nurse-guide
- Free shipping
- Aftercare integration and support

"From as low as $99/month" the site states, but again with an asterisk denoting "*With financing available through Walnut."

## WONDERMED

**Type of ketamine offered:** Racemic ketamine oral lozenge.

Wondermed (www.wondermed.com) offers low-dose, prescription oral ketamine treatment for patients to take at home. Treatment consists of 4+ Self-Led Ketamine Treatment Sessions including a consult with a clinician and access to other tools and resources such as a treatment kit and online support. Prices are cited as $319 (a new patient special at the time of writing, December 2022) and $399.

## PAIN CENTERS

A number of different pain centers, or clinics that specialize in treatments for chronic pain, may also offer ketamine treatment as one of their services. You may have to do a little searching to find these in your local town or city.

## PSYCHEDELIC SUPPORT

One of the greatest finds in the world of ketamine therapy is Psychedelic Support. Psychedelic Support has a provider search tool that allows you to look for providers that offer psychedelic therapies, including ketamine treatment; you can access it at psychedelic .support/network. You can also join local psychedelic community groups and search for psychedelic clinical trials there, too.

## BONUS: TRIP SITTER OPTIONS

If you are using ketamine at home and are a little anxious going through the journey alone, you can always hire a trip sitter. A trip sitter is an individual who is specially trained to comfort and guide people going through a psychedelic experience. One such service is Psychedelic Passage (www.psychedelicpassage.com).

# FINANCIAL ASSISTANCE OPTIONS

If insurance won't cover ketamine treatment, and you don't happen to have a couple of thousand dollars lying around, you may have to look into some creative financing options.

Some ketamine treatment centers offer discounts for especially vulnerable populations. Ketamine Wellness Centers (ketaminewellnesscenters.com), for instance, offer a Hero Discount for the following:

- Military personnel (Army, Navy, Air Force, Marine Corps, National Guard, Reserves, and Coast Guard)
- Police officers
- EMTs, paramedics
- Border patrol officers
- Correctional officers

Another provider, CIT Clinics (citclinics.com), offers free ketamine treatment to veterans in Northern California.

# ETHICAL CONCERNS OF TELEHEALTH SERVICES

As much as I want patients to have safe, easy access to ketamine therapy via telehealth services—I have to say there are some serious concerns to lay out here. Consider my experience completing an intake form for one telehealth provider:

"I don't see anything here that would disqualify you for treatment," Rogers, my Joyous nurse practitioner, says cheerily, as I sit on the other side of the screen with a smile frozen in place, desperate not to give anything away. You see, Joyous determines patient eligibility largely using online tools to collect information. While I completed an extensive intake form online before I was scheduled, great, big parts of this process sent up red flags.

Who, if anyone, was verifying the answers patients provided in their initial intake forms?

As I continued to navigate the form, I felt fear grow inside me. What if I accidentally answered yes to having a condition that was contra-indicated? This concern applied to nearly any telehealth program I wanted to try out. I did not know in advance which conditions each program considered to be contraindications; there was no list. And yet, if I was here because conventional medications and treatments had failed me—if I was truly in need and desperate—how could I possibly be motivated to tell the truth in a situation where it may hurt my chances for treatment? It's a sick game of trial and error.

It makes me wonder about patients with other conditions that may be contraindicated, such as bipolar disorder or schizophrenia. Could those patients, too, easily lie about symptoms to receive a drug that may or may not exacerbate their symptoms? Could criminals pretend to be patients in order to obtain drugs for nefarious purposes?

The potential for abuse here terrifies me. What can we do to make this a safer process for patients and providers?

# MDs VS NURSE PRACTITIONERS

Another thing to consider is the medical providers each program offers. Joyous, for instance, employs what is now an increasingly common practice of using nurse practitioners to assess patients. Redditers complained that the quality of care by Dr. Smith of the infamous Smith Family MD declined as he grew in popularity: "I know Dr. Smith. I have to say when he first started his practice, he would see every patient individually. Now that he has employed NPs [nurse practitioners] to see patients it seems like it's a conveyor belt."

Given all the facts, I can't help but feel MDs should be involved in this process, that leaving assessment and other vital features of ketamine treatment solely in the hands of nurse practitioners is irresponsible at best and dangerous at worst.

According to a working paper from the National Bureau of Economic Research, a study found that nurse practitioners use more resources but generate worse health outcomes than licensed physicians. Their results showed that nurse practitioners increased lengths of stay by 11 percent while elevating costs of emergency department visits by 7 percent. This amounts to an estimated 18-minute increase in the length of stay, and a $66 increase in cost for every emergency department visit (Chan and Chen 2022).

Ketamine is still an emerging mode of therapy. It's unique, complex, and highly dose dependent. A clear list of contraindications, information on dosing, and other safety concerns still has not been fully evaluated. Patients who may be experiencing negative side effects of the drug can also be very challenging to manage.

Given that information, I believe ketamine therapy is best left in the hands of the most well-trained professionals available.

# POTENTIAL FOR ABUSE

After browsing Reddit's r/TherapeuticKetamine subreddit, another concern began to roll around in my stomach regarding dosing and the potential for abuse.

"You get a pack of 30 lozenges five to seven business days after completing your telehealth appointment with a nurse practitioner," my Joyous nurse practitioner, Lexus Rogers, continued.

I never abused my take-home, oral ketamine treatment in Oregon; never once saved up a few days' doses and then took a very large recreational dose for fun. But some patients receiving at-home ketamine, however, did. I read several posts on r/TherapeuticKetamine in which people talked about saving up daily ketamine doses to take larger doses, or self-induce trips, later on.

Joyous also relies on AI software to manage patients' doses.

"All of your dosing is going to be done through the AI automation. These are text messages you're going to get every day where it's going to be asking questions about your mood, side effects you may be having, as well as tell you what your dose is going to be for that particular day," Rogers explained.

Now this sounds like a nice system on paper…provided everyone is honest and sticks to their daily dosing plan, of course. But sadly, humans have proven beyond a doubt that we simply do not deserve to have nice things. It would be all too easy, I fear, for any patient to lie about their symptom severity; for any patient to pretend they need a far larger dose than what was therapeutically advisable.

I have seen the therapeutic side of ketamine where this drug has saved lives. I have also known people that have destroyed their lives with it.

I cannot urge people enough: *please do not abuse ketamine.* Ketamine can be beneficial, yes, but it also comes with a number of side effects that require medical supervision. I can understand a patient in severe distress using microdoses on a daily basis for at-home treatment; there's little concern in that. But as we explained earlier, larger doses of ketamine can produce anything from increases in blood pressure, to psychosis, to full on "K-holes," which are decidedly *not* therapeutic and can even be dangerous.

This puts those in the therapeutic ketamine community in quite the pickle. How can we continue to advocate for easier access to ketamine therapies while also keeping practices ethical and maintaining patient safety? How do we create systems that keep abuse in check without reducing a patient's ability to get treatment?

Medical health professionals are still trying to figure out the answers to these questions.

# MIXING DRUGS

"How about a bump of ketamine after some beers?"

Ah, we've all been tempted, haven't we? A bump here, a keyhole there…

Now I don't mean to seem like your stern mama, but boy howdy, let me tell you: *do not mix ketamine with other drugs.*

I repeat for everyone in the back: DO NOT MIX KETAMINE WITH OTHER DRUGS. This includes alcohol *and* cannabis.

*Whaaaaat??? Be cool, man.*

No way, homeslice. Trust me, no one is a bigger advocate of drugs for therapeutic healing than yours truly. But mixing ketamine is not the way to do that. I say this based on extensive personal experience.

For starters, ketamine is a dissociative drug that has different effects depending on dosage. Small doses can be therapeutic—but larger doses can produce more sedating effects, including these listed by the US Department of Justice:

- mental confusion
- catalepsy (the inability to move)
- amnesia (memory loss)
- convulsions
- a delusional dream-like state
- hallucinations (auditory and visual)
- psychosis, or a loss of touch with reality

Since measuring a dose is almost impossible at the consumer level, there's no way for you to have any idea just how much ketamine you're consuming. Add some alcohol to the mix, and you have yourself a powerful tool for blacking out. Combining ketamine with alcohol was, incidentally, one of the DEA's reasons for banning ketamine as the two combined could be used to facilitate sexual assault:

> "Drugs being used by perpetrators in crimes of sexual assault include, but are not limited to, Rohypnol, GHB (Gamma Hydroxybutyric Acid), GBL (Gamma-Butyrolactone), and ketamine. In certain amounts, any drug can leave you helpless. These drugs are sometimes used by a perpetrator as a tactic to facilitate sexual assault because they have sedative effects."

Curious to learn more about the effects of ketamine and alcohol? Check out this research paper published in the 2022 *International*

*Journal of Molecular Sciences*: "Ketamine plus Alcohol: What We Know and What We Can Expect about This" (Kobayashi 2022).

*Ugh, okay. What about cannabis?*

The answer is still a solid, cool no, baby. And that's not because I don't approve of cannabis, either. Much like the case of alcohol and ketamine, combining ketamine with cannabis can increase certain effects that can be disorienting. You might discover, as I did early on when attempting this, that you have lost control of your limbs entirely. You might even find your limbs moving on their own, or other strange effects manifesting that can be downright unpleasant (and I say this as a VERY experienced cannabis user). This combination can also be especially dangerous for patients who may be genetically predisposed to certain conditions that entail psychosis, such as schizophrenia.

In short, wait a few hours after cannabis use before consuming ketamine, and vice versa (do not consume cannabis concurrently with ketamine). One notable (potential) exception to this rule is cannabidiol (CBD), a non-intoxicating cannabinoid derived from hemp. Recent studies have shown promising results with regard to CBD and ketamine administration. A paper published in the 2021 issue of *Neuropharmacology* found that administering CBD along with ketamine "induced significant dose-dependent antidepressant effects" (Sartim et al. 2021). Researchers concluded that CBD and ketamine's combined administration "can be a promising therapeutic strategy for achieving an appropriate antidepressant effect without unwanted side-effects."

Chapter 6

# KETAMINE: A NEW HOPE

By now you've learned about ketamine, its history, and its therapeutic promise. But just what are researchers today doing with this fascinating molecule? Let's check out what they've been up to. What does the future of ketamine hold? What's on the horizon, and what can we expect next?

## CURRENT MEDICAL CONDITIONS

As of December 2022, ketamine is currently being considered as a viable treatment option for a number of different conditions. These include the following:

- Depression (unipolar and bipolar)
- Major depressive disorder (MDD)
- Suicidal ideation/acute suicidality
- Obsessive compulsive disorder (OCD)
- Bipolar disorder
- Posttraumatic stress disorder (PTSD)
- Substance abuse/dependence
- Gambling disorders
- Autism spectrum disorder
- Parkinson's disease
- Ischemic stroke
- Fibromyalgia
- Eating disorders
- Neuropathic pain
- Fatigue
- Borderline personality disorder

While the data we do have regarding ketamine is promising, more controlled research is needed to determine its role in treating these conditions.

As more research unfolds, we will continue to learn more about ketamine's potential treatment options and limitations.

# KETAMINE AND BRAIN FUNCTION

Dr. Nazeer is currently working on gathering data and examining the clinical effects of ketamine when it comes to cognition. His clinic conducts objective, computer-based neurocognitive testing in all patients prior to starting ketamine treatment, as well as at intervals after initial administration.

"We've been collecting data for some years and we will be looking to see what kind of clinical correlations we see with brain function and cognition related to ketamine," says Dr. Nazeer. Nazeer's team is also evaluating outcome data to see "what clinical pearls and insights we can gain based on different diagnoses and patient types, different doses of ketamine, different schedules of ketamine maintenance."

As the study of ketamine and its effects on brain function continues, researchers hope to uncover a greater understanding of the true therapeutic potential of this powerful compound. With the potential to provide relief from a range of conditions from depression to Parkinson's disease, the scientific community—and patients everywhere—are eager to explore the full extent of ketamine's capabilities.

# PREVENTING PTSD

As noted, ketamine may be useful in preventing the development of PTSD. This represents another exciting avenue for ketamine exploration, especially with respect to critically vulnerable populations.

"Future direction for research is to examine how ketamine can be used—not as a treatment for pathology, but as a protective prior treatment for professionals at risk of PTSD," says Mitchell. He draws on the hope that ketamine will begin to treat veterans, enlisted soldiers, addicts, and suicidal populations—those who need it most—first.

"First responders, police, and child abuse investigators are all populations who, encountering a great amount of observed trauma in their work, are at risk of acquiring PTSD far beyond lay populations," Mitchell says. "The way ketamine affects our corticosteroid hormone system shows a protective capacity for these populations." He suggests the idea that ketamine can be given to especially vulnerable populations out in the field to help mitigate any potential trauma, and, in turn, halt PTSD in its tracks. Red Cross workers, for instance, could be administered ketamine before missions, making them less likely to take trauma home with them.

"Ketamine may not be able to eliminate trauma, but the ways it can reduce it are just now beginning to be understood," Mitchell adds. Researchers are currently evaluating ketamine's ability to reduce PTSD symptoms in veterans and service members with PTSD that had been failed by previous antidepressant treatments (Abdallah et al. 2022)

# REMOTE ACCESS TO DOSING

One major hurdle in the world of ketamine therapy is a lack of trained clinical professionals who can supervise patients during administration.

The ketamine microneedle patch pioneered by PharmaTher, KETABET™ MN, uses hydrogel-forming microneedle arrays to "overcome any limitations by the quantity of drug that can be loaded into the needles or onto the needle surfaces" (Newscope Capital Corporation 2021). The end result is a greater amount of ketamine that can permeate through skin.

KETABET™ MN will also include anti-tampering and anti-abuse features so patients can safely dose themselves remotely rather than having to be under supervision of a medical professional.

The implementation of new technology in health care is often influenced by a number of factors including cost, reimbursement, and overall convenience for both patients and providers. Therefore, the integration of technology like KETABET™ MN into health-care clinics and for use by patients will likely depend on a number of factors including the results of clinical trials, regulatory approval, and overall market demand.

Before a new product like KETABET™ MN can be widely used, it must undergo rigorous clinical testing to demonstrate its safety and efficacy. This can take several years and may involve multiple phases of clinical trials. Once a product has undergone testing and been approved by regulatory bodies, such as the FDA, it is likely that health-care providers will begin to incorporate it into their clinics and make it available to patients.

It's also important to note that the timeline for the widespread use of products like KETABET™ MN will depend on the results of ongoing clinical trials and regulatory approval. At this time, it is difficult to predict exactly when patients will be able to access this technology and begin to see its integration into health care.

# KETAMINE AND LOU GEHRIG'S DISEASE

In January 2022, PharmaTher, a Canadian company and "leader in specialty ketamine pharmaceuticals," received FDA approval to proceed with a phase II clinical trial employing use of ketamine to treat amyotrophic lateral sclerosis (ALS), also known as Lou Gehrig's disease (Microdose Psychedelic Insights 2022). Lou Gehrig's disease is a type of neurodegenerative disease in which neurons controlling voluntary movement are attacked.

Some preclinical studies have shown that low-dose ketamine treatment can reduce oxidative stress and inflammation, improve motor function, and delay the progression of ALS-like symptoms in animal models (Stanford et al. 2021).

It's important to note that these findings are based on animal studies. More research is ultimately needed to determine the safety and efficacy of ketamine in humans with ALS.

# KETAMINE AND EPILEPSY

Researchers are interested in assessing ketamine's ability to play a role in the treatment of several neurological conditions. A medication developed by PharmaTher was granted "orphan drug" status by the FDA in February of 2022 to treat status epilepticus, a prolonged type of seizure that can be life threatening (Microdose Psychedelic Insights 2022). Orphan drug designation is issued by the FDA for "supporting the development and evaluation of new treatments for rare diseases."

PharmaTher's orphan drug portfolio, incidentally, already includes the use of ketamine to treat Lou Gehrig's disease as well as complex regional pain syndrome. The company also noted that their most recent orphan drug designation strengthens their ability to expand on the development of novel ketamine delivery methods such as a microneedle patch for other rare conditions.

# KETAMINE AND PARKINSON'S DISEASE

On July 13, 2022, PharmaTher was granted a Notice of Allowance for a new, novel ketamine patent designed to employ ketamine for the potential treatment of Parkinson's disease.

PharmaTher is currently planning a phase III clinical study to get FDA approval of their proprietary intravenous ketamine product, KETARX™ (Najum 2022).

Ketamine is a promising treatment option for Parkinson's disease due to its ability to affect certain neurotransmitter systems in the brain that are involved in the regulation of movement.

Parkinson's is characterized by a degeneration of dopamine-producing cells in the brain, which leads to symptoms such as tremors, stiffness, and difficulty with movement and coordination.

Ketamine's ability to stimulate the release of glutamate can lead to improvements in symptoms of Parkinson's. Intravenous forms of ketamine such as KETARX™ have the potential to provide rapid and more effective relief compared to oral forms of the drug.

PharmaTher's phase III clinical study for KETARX™ is an important step in obtaining FDA approval for the use of intravenous ketamine as a treatment for Parkinson's. If successful, this study will provide evidence of the safety and efficacy of the drug, which may lead to its widespread use in treating Parkinson's patients.

It is important to note that while ketamine has shown promise as a treatment for Parkinson's, more research is needed to fully understand its effects and determine the best dosing and administration methods. Additionally, while KETARX™ has been granted a Notice of Allowance for a new, novel ketamine patent, it is still in the process of undergoing clinical trials and has not yet been approved by the FDA for use in the treatment of Parkinson's disease.

# KAP IMPLICATIONS

Another promising way ketamine can shape the world is by debunking outdated models of approaching conditions like depression. The idea of depression as an imbalance of hormones needing correction is ebbing away in favor of a new model focused on introspection and cognitive expansion.

"The current standard of care is to diagnose a disease state and provide an algorithmic treatment option consisting mainly of daily medication," Dr. Zand explains. "We are hopeful that the diagnostic criteria of mental illness will shift toward a more broad self-exploration and mind-expansion paradigm. Removing the current labels in mental health and refocusing our intentions on improved brain function and subconscious reprogramming, we will see a vast improvement in mental health care."

Researchers are already beginning to test out the ways in which ketamine's neuroplastic effects can be prolonged, too. A study published in *American Journal of Psychiatry* found that the antidepressant effects of ketamine could be extended long after treatment with a few simple tweaks (Price et al. 2022).

Hoping to capitalize on ketamine's neuroplasticity window, Price's team of researchers had test subjects play computer games after receiving ketamine. These weren't just any computer games, however; they were games focused on improving participants' sense of self-esteem and decreasing their sense of self-loathing. Games that involved words, for instance, paired positive terms like "good," "lovable," "sweet," "worthy," etc., every time a participant saw the word "I." The end result?

"By doing these really simple computer exercises we could extend the antidepressant effect of one infusion of ketamine for at least a month," says Rebecca Price, an author of the study and an associate professor of psychiatry and psychology at the University of Pittsburgh.

Participants in the study remained free of depression for periods of up to three months following ketamine infusions. In contrast, patients who received infusions without computer games tended to relapse after a week or two.

This study is also especially promising as it introduces the concept of automated, computerized elements to ketamine therapy—and health-care professionals are in short supply. Dr. Sanjay Mathew, a coauthor of the study and professor of psychiatry at Baylor College of Medicine, also adds that if these results are maintained in larger studies, it may significantly reduce the cost of ketamine therapy moving forward (Hamilton 2022).

# CONCLUSION

If you're still here with me: thank you for your time, effort, and love. It's been a privilege to share this information with you, and I'm honored to have you as my audience.

I hope you've learned a thing or two from these pages, and I hope that can help you with whatever you ail from.

The world of ketamine is growing rapidly, so much so that I continued to discover new research every day even as I was writing this book.

I can't wait to see what comes next.

# BIBLIOGRAPHY

Abdallah, C. G., et al. "Dose-Related Effects of Ketamine for Antidepressant-Resistant Symptoms of Posttraumatic Stress Disorder in Veterans and Active Duty Military: A Double-Blind, Randomized, Placebo-Controlled Multi-Center Clinical Trial." *Neuropsychopharmacology* 47, no. 8 (2022): 1574–81, doi: 10.1038/s41386-022-01266-9.

Abdallah, C. G., et al. "Ketamine's Mechanism of Action: A Path to Rapid-Acting Antidepressants." *Depression and Anxiety* 33, no. 8 (2017): 689–697, doi: 10.1002/da.22501.

Abdallah, C. G., et al. "Prefrontal Cortical GABA Abnormalities Are Associated with Reduced Hippocampal Volume in Major Depressive Disorder." *European Neuropsychopharmacology* 25, no. 8 (2015): 1082–1090, doi: 10.1016/j.euroneuro.2015.04.025.

Abraham, H. D., A. M. Aldridge, and P. Gogia. "The Psychopharmacology of Hallucinogens." *Neuropsychopharmacology* 14, no. 4 (1996): 285–98, doi: 10.1016/0893-133X(95)00136-2.

Albanèse, J., S. Arnaud, M. Rey, L. Thomachot, B. Alliez, and C. Martin. "Ketamine Decreases Intracranial Pressure and Electroencephalographic Activity in Traumatic Brain Injury Patients during Propofol Sedation." *Anesthesiology* 87, no. 6 (1997): 1328–34, doi: 10.1097/00000542-199712000-00011.

Backman, Isabella. "Ketamine: Handle with Care." Medicine.yale.edu. April 10, 2023. medicine.yale.edu/news-article/ketamine-handle-with-care.

Bahji, A., G. H. Vazquez, and C. A. Zarate, Jr. "Comparative Efficacy of Racemic Ketamine and Esketamine for Depression: A Systematic Review and Meta-Analysis." *Journal of Affective Disorders* 278 (2021): 12473, doi: 10.1016/j.jad.2020.09.071.

Ballantyne, J. C. "Chapter 17–Complications Associated with Systemic Opioids and Patient-Controlled Analgesia." *Complications in Regional Anesthesia & Pain Medicine* (2007): 167–75. www.sciencedirect.com/science/article/pii/B9781416023920500212.

Bar-Joseph, G., Y. Guilburd, A. Tamir, and J. N. Guilburd. "Effectiveness of Ketamine in Decreasing Intracranial Pressure in Children with Intracranial Hypertension." *Journal of Neurosurgery: Pediatrics* 4, no. 1 (2009): 40–46, doi: 10.3171/2009.1.peds08319.

Berman, R. M., A. Cappiello, A. Anand, D. A. Oren, G. R. Heninger, D. S. Charney, and J. H. Krystal. "Antidepressant Effects of Ketamine in Depressed Patients." *Biolological Psychiatry* 47, no. 4 (2000): 351-54, doi: 10.1016/s0006-3223(99)00230-9.

Bibi, Z. "Role of Cytochrome P450 in Drug Interactions." *Nutrition & Metabolism* 5, no. 1 (2008): 27, doi: 10.1186/1743-7075-5-27.

Bloch, M. H., et al. "Effects of Ketamine in Treatment-Refractory Obsessive-Compulsive Disorder." *Biological Psychiatry* 72, no. 11 (2012): 964–970, doi: 10.1016/j.biopsych.2012.05.028.

Bonson, K. R. "Regulation of Human Research with LSD in the United States (1949–1987)." *Psychopharmacology* 235, no. 2 (2018): 591–604, doi: 10.1007/s00213-017-4777-4.

Bowdle, A. T., A. D. Radant, D. S. Cowley, E. D. Kharasch, R. J. Strassman, and P. P. Roy-Byrne. "Psychedelic Effects of Ketamine in Healthy Volunteers." *Anesthesiology* 88, no. 1 (1998): 82–88, doi: 10.1097/00000542-199801000-00015.

Brachman, R. A., et al. "Ketamine as a Prophylactic against Stress-Induced Depressive-like Behavior." *Biological Psychiatry* 79, no. 9 (2016): 776–86, doi: 10.1016/j.biopsych.2015.04.022.

Breeksema, J. J., et al. "Holding on or Letting Go? Patient Experiences of Control, Context, and Care in Oral Esketamine Treatment for Treatment-Resistant Depression: A Qualitative Study." *Frontiers in Psychiatry* 13 (2022): doi: 10.3389/fpsyt.2022.948115.

Brooks, Kayla. "People Seeking Mental Health Treatment Navigate Long Wait Times." WHSV.com. March 3, 2022. https://www.whsv.com/2022/03/04/people-seeking-mental-health-treatment-navigate-long-wait-times.

Brown, R. H., and E. M. Wagner. "Mechanisms of Bronchoprotection by Anesthetic Induction Agents: Propofol versus Ketamine." *Anesthesiology* 90, no. 3 (1999): 822–28, doi: 10.1097/00000542-199903000-00025.

Buckner, R. L. "The Brain's Default Network: Origins and Implications for the Study of Psychosis." *Dialogues in Clinical Neuroscience* 15, no. 3 (2013): 351–58, doi: 10.31887/DCNS.2013.15.3/rbuckner.

Canuso, C. M., et al. "Efficacy and Safety of Intranasal Esketamine for the Rapid Reduction of Symptoms of Depression and Suicidality in Patients at Imminent Risk for Suicide: Results of a Double-Blind, Randomized,

Placebo-Controlled Study." *American Journal of Psychiatry* 175, no. 7
(2018): 620–30, doi: 10.1176/appi.ajp.2018.17060720.

Capuzzi, Enrico, et al. "Long-Term Efficacy of Intranasal Esketamine
in Treatment-Resistant Major Depression: A Systematic Review."
*International Journal of Molecular Sciences* 22, no. 17 (August 28, 2021):
9338. doi: 10.3390/ijms22179338.

Carey, Benedict. "Fast-Acting Depression Drug, Newly Approved, Could Help
Millions." *New York Times*. March 6, 2019. www.nytimes.com/2019/03/05
/health/depression-treatment-ketamine-fda.html.

Carhart-Harris, R. L., and G. M. Goodwin. "The Therapeutic Potential of
Psychedelic Drugs: Past, Present, and Future." *Neuropsychopharmacology*
42, no. 11 (2017): 2105–13, doi: 10.1038/npp.2017.84.

Carrion, Victor G., et al. "Converging Evidence for Abnormalities of the
Prefrontal Cortex and Evaluation of Midsagittal Structures in Pediatric
Posttraumatic Stress Disorder: An MRI Study." *Psychiatry Research:
Neuroimaging* 172, no. 3 (June 2009): 226–34. doi: 10.1016/j.pscychresns
.2008.07.008.

Center for Drug Evaluation and Research. "Frequently Asked Questions about
the FDA Drug Approval Process." FDA. February 9, 2019. www.fda.gov
/drugs/special-features/frequently-asked-questions-about-fda-drug
-approval-process#4.

Chan, Jr., David C., and Yiqun Chen. "The Productivity of Professions:
Evidence from the Emergency Department." *National Bureau of Economic
Research*. October 1, 2022. www.nber.org/papers/w30608.

Chu, Andrew, and Roopma Wadhwa. "Selective Serotonin Reuptake
Inhibitors." PubMed, StatPearls Publishing, 2021, www.ncbi.nlm.nih.gov
/books/NBK554406/.

Clements, J. A., W. S. Nimmo, and I. S. Grant. "Bioavailability,
Pharmacokinetics, and Analgesic Activity of Ketamine in Humans."
*Journal of Pharmaceutical Sciences* 71, no. 5 (1982): 539–42, doi: 10.1002
/jps.2600710516.

"Clinical Practice Guidelines: Ketamine Use for Procedural Sedation." rch.org
.au. Last updated December 2021. www.rch.org.au/clinicalguide
/guideline_index/Ketamine_use_for_procedural_sedation.

Collo, G., and E. M. Pich. "Ketamine Enhances Structural Plasticity in Human
Dopaminergic Neurons: Possible Relevance for Treatment-Resistant
Depression." *Neural Regeneration Research* 13, no. 4 (2018): 645, doi:
10.4103/1673-5374.230288.

Corkery, J. M., W. Hung, and F. Schifano. "Recreational Ketamine-Related Deaths Notified to the National Programme on Substance Abuse Deaths, England, 1997–2019." *Journal of Psychopharmacology* 35, no. 11 (2021): 1324-48, doi: 10.1177/02698811211021588.

Corssen G., and E. F. Domino. "Dissociative Anesthesia: Further Pharmacologic Studies and First Clinical Experience with the Phencyclidine Derivative CI-581." *Anesthesia & Analgesia* 45 (1966): 29–40, doi: 10.1213/00000539-196601000-00007.

Cui, Y., S. Hu, and H. Hu. "Lateral Habenular Burst Firing as a Target of the Rapid Antidepressant Effects of Ketamine." *Trends in Neurosciences* 42, no. 3 (2019): 179–91, doi: 10.1016/j.tins.2018.12.002.

D'Andrea, D., and R. A. Sewell. "Transient Resolution of Treatment-Resistant Posttraumatic Stress Disorder Following Ketamine Infusion." *Biological Psychiatry* 74, no. 9 (2013): e13–e14, doi: 10.1016/j.biopsych.2013.04.019.

Dakwar, E., et al. "A Single Ketamine Infusion Combined with Motivational Enhancement Therapy for Alcohol Use Disorder: A Randomized Midazolam-Controlled Pilot Trial." *American Journal of Psychiatry* 177, no. 2 (2019): 125–33, doi: 10.1176/appi.ajp.2019.19070684.

Dakwar, E., F. Levin, R. W. Foltin, E. V. Nunes, and C. L. Hart. "The Effects of Subanesthetic Ketamine Infusions on Motivation to Quit and Cue-Induced Craving in Cocaine-Dependent Research Volunteers." *Biological Psychiatry* 76, no. 1 (2014): 40–46, doi: 10.1016/j.biopsych.2013.08.009.

Daly, Ella J., et al. "Efficacy of Esketamine Nasal Spray plus Oral Antidepressant Treatment for Relapse Prevention in Patients with Treatment-Resistant Depression." *JAMA Psychiatry* 76, no. 9 (June 5 2019). doi: 10.1001/jamapsychiatry.2019.1189.

David, D., et al. "Why Cognitive Behavioral Therapy Is the Current Gold Standard of Psychotherapy." *Frontiers in Psychiatry* 9, no. 4 (2018): 1–3, doi: 10.3389/fpsyt.2018.00004.

"Depression." *World Health Organization*. September 13, 2021. www.who.int /news-room/fact-sheets/detail/depression.

Diana, M., J. Quilez, and M. Rafecas. "Gamma-Aminobutyric Acid as a Bioactive Compound in Foods: A Review." *Journal of Functional Foods* 10 (2014): 407–20, doi: 10.1016/j.jff.2014.07.004.

Diazgranados, N., et al. "A Randomized Add-on Trial of an N-Methyl-D-Aspartate Antagonist in Treatment-Resistant Bipolar Depression." *Archives of General Psychiatry* 67, no. 8 (2010): 793, doi: 10.1001/archgenpsychiatry .2010.90.

THE KETAMINE HANDBOOK

Domino, Edward F. "History and Pharmacology of PCP and PCP-Related Analogs." *Journal of Psychedelic Drugs* 12, no. 3-4 (1980): 223–27, doi: 10.1080/02791072.1980.10471430.

Domino, E. F., P. Chodoff, and G. Corssen. "Pharmacologic Effects of CI-581, a New Dissociative Anesthetic, in Man." *Clinical Pharmacology & Therapeutics* 6, no. 3 (1965): 279–91, doi: 10.1002/cpt196563279.

Dong, T. T., et al. "Ketamine: A Growing Global Health-Care Need." *British Journal of Anaesthesia* 115, no. 4 (2015): 491–93, doi: 10.1093/bja/aev215.

Dore, J., et al. "Ketamine Assisted Psychotherapy (KAP): Patient Demographics, Clinical Data and Outcomes in Three Large Practices Administering Ketamine with Psychotherapy." *Journal of Psychoactive Drugs* 51, no. 2 (2019): 189–98, doi: 10.1080/02791072.2019.1587556.

Duman, R. S., and L. M. Monteggia. "A Neurotrophic Model for Stress-Related Mood Disorders." *Biological Psychiatry* 59, no. 12 (2006): 1116–27, doi: 10.1016/j.biopsych.2006.02.013.

Drug Enforcement Administration. "Drug Scheduling." DEA.gov. July 10, 2018. www.dea.gov/drug-information/drug-scheduling.

Drug Enforcement Administration. Part 520—Oral Dosage Form New Animal Drugs. www.govinfo.gov/content/pkg/FR-1999-07-13/pdf/99-17803.pdf.

Drug Enforcement Administration. "Schedules of Controlled Substances: Placement of Ketamine into Schedule III." *Federal Register* 64, no, 133 (199): 37673. https://www.govinfo.gov/content/pkg/FR-1999-07-13/pdf /99-17803.pdf.

Drug Enforcement Administration. "What Is Ketamine?" April 2020. www.dea .gov/sites/default/files/2020-06/Ketamine-2020.pdf.

Eikermann, M., et al. "Ketamine Activates Breathing and Abolishes the Coupling between Loss of Consciousness and Upper Airway Dilator Muscle Dysfunction." *Anesthesiology* 116, no. 1 (2012): 35–46, doi: 10.1097/aln .0b013e31823d010a.

Fava, Giovanni A. "May Antidepressant Drugs Worsen the Conditions They Are Supposed to Treat? The Clinical Foundations of the Oppositional Model of Tolerance." *Therapeutic Advances in Psychopharmacology* 10 (2020). doi: 10.1177/2045125320970325.

"FDA Approves Medication Related to Party-Drug 'Special K' in First Major Depression Treatment to Hit Market in Decades." *Kaiser Health News*. March 6, 2019. https://khn.org/morning-breakout /fda-approves-medication-related-to-party-drug-special-k-in-first-major -depression-treatment-to-hit-market-in-decades.

"FDA Overlooked Red Flags in Testing of New Depression Drug." *The Daily Beast*. Last updated June 10, 2019. www.thedailybeast.com/fda-overlooked-red-flags-while-testing-new-depression-drug-it-approved.

Feder, A., et al. "Efficacy of Intravenous Ketamine for Treatment of Chronic Posttraumatic Stress Disorder." *JAMA Psychiatry* 71, no. 6 (2014): 681, doi: 10.1001/jamapsychiatry.2014.62.

Ferguson, J. M. "SSRI Antidepressant Medications: Adverse Effects and Tolerability." *Primary Care Companion to the Journal of Clinical Psychiatry* 3, no. 1 (2001): 22–27. www.ncbi.nlm.nih.gov/pmc/articles/PMC181155.

Fork (contributor). Review of *Journeys into the Bright World*, by Marcia Moore and Howard Alltounian. August 21, 2012. erowid.org/library/review/review.php?p=360.

Gahlinger, P. M. "Club Drugs: MDMA, Gamma-Hydroxybutyrate (GHB), Rohypnol, and Ketamine." *American Family Physician* 69, no. 11 (2004): 2619–26, doi: 10.4088/pcc.v03n0105.

Gamo, N. J., and A. F. T. Arnsten. "Molecular Modulation of Prefrontal Cortex: Rational Development of Treatments for Psychiatric Disorders." *Behavioral Neuroscience* 125, no. 3 (2011): 282–96, doi: 10.1037/a0023165.

Gayhart, Susan. "Explaining My Experiences with Ketamine for Those Considering Ketamine Therapy." Boise Ketamine Clinic. January 28, 2019. boiseketamineclinic.com/my-ketamine-story-explaining-my-experiences-with-ketamine-for-those-considering-ketamine-therapy.

Gold, P. W., and B. Kadriu. "A Major Role for the Lateral Habenula in Depressive Illness: Physiologic and Molecular Mechanisms." *Frontiers in Psychiatry: Molecular Psychiatry* 10 (2019): 320, doi: 10.3389/fpsyt.2019.00320.

Goldhill, Olivia. "Ketamine's Promise as an Antidepressant Is Being Undermined by Its Lack of Profit." Yahoo Finance. August 6, 2020. www.yahoo.com/video/ketamine-promise-antidepressant-being-undermined-181000304.html.

Grant, J. E., and S. R. Chamberlain. "Response of Refractory Gambling Disorder to Intravenous Ketamine." *The Primary Care Companion for CNS Disorders* 22, no. 1 (2020), 19l02480, doi: 10.4088/pcc.19l02480.

Greifenstein, F. E., M. Devault, J. Yoshitake, and J. E. Gajewski. "A Study of A 1-Aryl Cyclo Hexyl Amine For Anesthesia." *Anesthesia & Analgesia* 37, no. 5 (1958): 283–94, doi: 13583607.

Gregers, M. C. T., et al. "Ketamine as an Anesthetic for Patients with Acute Brain Injury: A Systematic Review." *Neurocritical Care* 33, no. 1 (2020): 273–82, doi: 10.1007/s12028-020-00975-7.

Grof, Stanislav. *LSD Psychotherapy*. Ben Lomond, CA: Multidisciplinary Association for Psychedelic Studies, 2008.

Guimarães Pereira, L. F. G. Pereira, R. M. Linhares, C. D. A. Bersot, T. Aslanidis, and H. A. Ashmawi. "Efficacy and Safety of Ketamine in the Treatment of Neuropathic Pain: A Systematic Review and Meta-Analysis of Randomized Controlled Trials." *Journal of Pain Research* 15 (2022): 1011–37, doi: 10.2147/jpr.s358070.

Hamilton, Jon. "Smiling Faces Might Help the Drug Ketamine Keep Depression at Bay." *NPR*. October 31, 2022. www.npr.org/sections/health -shots/2022/10/31/1132371480/smiling-faces-might-help-the-drug -ketamine-keep-depression-at-bay?utm_source=pocket_reader.

Hartogsohn, I. "The Meaning-Enhancing Properties of Psychedelics and Their Mediator Role in Psychedelic Therapy, Spirituality, and Creativity." *Frontiers in Neuroscience* 12 (2018), doi: 10.3389/fnins.2018.00129.

Hendrix, Steve. "Ketamine, a New Antidepressant, Has Been Blowing Minds for Decades." *Washington Post*. March 7, 2019. www.washingtonpost.com /history/2019/03/07/ketamine-new-anti-depressant-has-been-blowing- minds-decades.

Hepsomali, P., J. A. Groeger, J. Nishihira, and A. Scholey. "Effects of Oral Gamma-Aminobutyric Acid (GABA) Administration on Stress and Sleep in Humans: A Systematic Review." *Frontiers in Neuroscience* 14 (2020): 923, doi: 10.3389/fnins.2020.00923.

Hermle, L., et al. "Mescaline-Induced Psychopathological, Neuropsychological, and Neurometabolic Effects in Normal Subjects: Experimental Psychosis as a Tool for Psychiatric Research." *Biological Psychiatry* 32, no. 11 (1992): 976–91, doi: 10.1016/0006-3223(92)90059-9.

Hornik, C. P., et al. "Population Pharmacokinetics of Intramuscular and Intravenous Ketamine in Children." *The Journal of Clinical Pharmacology* 58, no. 8 (2018): 1092–1104, doi: 10.1002/jcph.1116.

Huetteman, Emmarie. "FDA Overlooked Red Flags in Drugmaker's Testing of New Depression Medicine." Kaiser Health News. June 11, 2019. khn.org /news/fdas-approval-of-new-depression-drug-overlooked-red-flags-in-its -testing.

Huetteman, Emmarie, and Kaiser Health News. "Ketamine-like Drug for Depression May Be Riskier than FDA Thought." *NBC News*. June 11, 2019. www.nbcnews.com/health/health-news/caution-urged-over-use-fast -acting-version-ketamine-depression-n1016176.

Hull, T. D., et al. "At-Home, Sublingual Ketamine Telehealth Is a Safe and Effective Treatment for Moderate to Severe Anxiety and Depression:

Findings from a Large, Prospective, Open-Label Effectiveness Trial." *Journal of Affective Disorders* 314 (2022): 59–67, doi: 10.1016 /j.jad.2022.07.004.

Irwin, S. A., A. Iglewicz, R. A. Nelesen, J. Y. Lo, C. H. Carr, S. D. Romero, and L. S. Lloyd. "Daily Oral Ketamine for the Treatment of Depression and Anxiety in Patients Receiving Hospice Care: A 28-Day Open-Label Proof-of -Concept Trial." *Journal of Palliative Medicine* 16, no. 8 (2013): 958–65, doi: 10.1089/jpm.2012.0617.

Jansen, Karl L. R. *Ketamine: Dreams and Realities*. Sarasota, FL: Multidisciplinary Association for Psychedelic Studies, 2004.

Janssen Pharmaceutical Companies of Johnson & Johnson. "Janssen Announces U.S. FDA Approval of SPRAVATO® (Esketamine) CIII Nasal Spray to Treat Depressive Symptoms in Adults with Major Depressive Disorder with Acute Suicidal Ideation or Behavior." PR Newswire. August 3, 2020. www.prnewswire.com/news-releases/janssen-announces-us-fda -approval-of-spravato-esketamine-ciii-nasal-spray-to-treat-depressive -symptoms-in-adults-with-major-depressive-disorder-with-acute-suicidal -ideation-or-behavior-301104437.html.

Janssen Research & Development, LLC. "A Randomized, Double-Blind, Multicenter, Active-Controlled Study of Intranasal Esketamine Plus An Oral Antidepressant for Relapse Prevention in Treatment-Resistant Depression." Clinicaltrials.gov. Last updated June 2, 2020. clinicaltrials. gov/ct2/show/study/NCT02493868.

Johnson & Johnson. "Janssen Announces U.S. FDA Approval of SPRAVATOTM (Esketamine) CIII Nasal Spray for Adults with Treatment-Resistant Depression (TRD) Who Have Cycled through Multiple Treatments without Relief." March 5, 2019. https://www.jnj.com/janssen-announces-u-s-fda -approval-of-spravatotm-esketamine-ciii-nasal-spray-for-adults-with -treatment-resistant-depression-trd-who-have-cycled-through-multiple -treatments-without-relief.

Johnstone, M., et al. "Sernyl (C1-395) In Clinical Anaesthesia." *British Journal of Anaesthesia* 31, no. 10 (1959): 433–39, doi: 10.1093/bja/31.10.433.

Joseph, T. T., et al. "Ketamine Metabolite (2$R$,6$R$)-Hydroxynorketamine Interacts with μ and κ Opioid Receptors." *ACS Chemical Neuroscience* 12, no. 9 (2021): 1487–97, doi: 10.1021/acschemneuro.0c00741.

Kabil, Ahmed. "The History of Psychedelics and Psychotherapy." Timeline. January 13, 2016. https://timeline.com/the-history-of-psychedelics-and -psychotherapy-fe70f72557aa.

Kassem, M. S., et al. "Stress-Induced Grey Matter Loss Determined by MRI Is Primarily due to Loss of Dendrites and Their Synapses." *Molecular Neurobiology* 47, no. 2 (2013): 645–61, doi: 10.1007/s12035-012-8365-7.

Kastner, T. A., K. Walsh, L. H. Shulman, F. Alam, and S. Flood. "Ketamine and the Core Symptoms of Autism." *International Journal on Disability and Human Development* 15, no. 1 (2016): 121–23, doi: 10.1515/ijdhd-2015 -0003.

Kempton, M. J. "Structural Neuroimaging Studies in Major Depressive Disorder." *Archives of General Psychiatry* 68, no. 7 (2011): 675, doi: 10.1001 /archgenpsychiatry.2011.60.

"Ketamine." DEA.gov. https://www.dea.gov/factsheets/ketamine.

Kirsch, I. "Antidepressants and the Placebo Effect." *Zeitschrift Für Psychologie* 222, no. 3 (2014): 128–34, doi: 10.1027/2151-2604/a000176.

Kobayashi, N. H. C., et al. "Ketamine plus Alcohol: What We Know and What We Can Expect about This." *International Journal of Molecular Sciences* 23, no. 14 (2022): 7800, doi: 10.3390/ijms23147800.

Kopra, E., et al. "Ketamine's Effect on Inflammation and Kynurenine Pathway in Depression: A Systematic Review." *Journal of Psychopharmacology* 35, no. 8 (2021): 934–45, doi: 10.1177/02698811211026426.

Krekow, Sylvie. "Ketamine Experiences: Would I Be in an Unfamiliar Environment with Unfamiliar People? And What If I Have a "Bad Trip"?" HealingMaps. April 8, 2022. healingmaps.com/personal-stories-ketamine.

Krupitsky, E. M., and A. Y. Grinenko. "Ketamine Psychedelic Therapy (KPT): A Review of the Results of Ten Years of Research." *Journal of Psychoactive Drugs* 29, no. 2 (1997): 165–83, doi: 10.1080/02791072.1997.10400185.

Krystal, John H. "Subanesthetic Effects of the Noncompetitive NMDA Antagonist, Ketamine, in Humans." *Archives of General Psychiatry* 51, no. 3 (1994): 199, doi: 10.1001/archpsyc.1994.03950030035004.

Krystal, J. H., et al. "Antidepressant Effects of Ketamine in Depressed Patients." *Biological Psychiatry* 4, no. 4 (2000): 351–54, doi: 10.1016 /s0006-3223(99)00230-9.

Krystal, J. H., et al. "Association of Combined Naltrexone and Ketamine with Depressive Symptoms in a Case Series of Patients with Depression and Alcohol Use Disorder." *JAMA Psychiatry* 76, no. 3 (2019): 337–38, doi: 10.1001/jamapsychiatry.2018.3990.

Langmia, I. M., K. S. Just, S. Yamounem, J. P. Muller, and J. C. Stingl. "Pharmacogenetic and Drug Interaction Aspects on Ketamine Safety in Its Use as Antidepressant–Implications for Precision Dosing in a Global

Perspective." *British Journal of Clinical Pharmacology* 88, no. 12 (2022): 5149–65, doi: 10.1111/bcp.15467.

Larkin, G. L., and A. L. Beautrais. "A Preliminary Naturalistic Study of Low-Dose Ketamine for Depression and Suicide Ideation in the Emergency Department." *International Journal of Neuropsychopharmacology* 14, no. 8 (2011): 1127–31, doi: 10.1017/s1461145711000629.

Laskowski, K., A. Stirling, W. P. McKay, and H. J. Lim. "A Systematic Review of Intravenous Ketamine for Postoperative Analgesia." *Canadian Journal of Anesthesia/Journal Canadien D'anesthésie* 58, no. 10 (2011): 911–23, doi: 10.1007/s12630-011-9560-0.

Lester, H. A., L. D. Lavis, and D. A. Dougherty. "Ketamine inside Neurons?" *The American Journal of Psychiatry* 172, no. 11 (2015): 1064–66, doi: 10.1176/appi.ajp.2015.14121537.

Li, Linda, and Phillip E Vlisides. "Ketamine: 50 Years of Modulating the Mind." *Frontiers in Human Neuroscience* 10 (Nov. 29, 2016): 612, doi: 10.3389/fnhum.2016.00612.

Li, N., et al. "MTOR-Dependent Synapse Formation Underlies the Rapid Antidepressant Effects of NMDA Antagonists." *Science* 329, no. 5994 (2010): 959–64, doi: 10.1126/science.1190287.

Liebe, T., et al. "Factors Influencing the Cardiovascular Response to Subanesthetic Ketamine: A Randomized, Placebo-Controlled Trial." *International Journal of Neuropsychopharmacology* 20, no. 11 (2017): 909–18, doi: 10.1093/ijnp/pyx055.

Liu, L., H. Huang, Y. Li, R. Zhang, Y. Wei, and W. Wu. "Severe Encephalatrophy and Related Disorders from Long-Term Ketamine Abuse: A Case Report and Literature Review." *Frontiers in Psychiatry* 12 (2021), doi: 10.3389/fpsyt.2021.707326.

Loo, C. K., et al. "Placebo-Controlled Pilot Trial Testing Dose Titration and Intravenous, Intramuscular and Subcutaneous Routes for Ketamine in Depression." *Acta Psychiatrica Scandinavica* 134, no. 1 (March 2016): 48–56. doi: 10.1111/acps.12572.

Malinovsky, J. M., et al. "Ketamine and Norketamine Plasma Concentrations after I.v., Nasal and Rectal Administration in Children." *British Journal of Anaesthesia* 77, no. 2 (1996): 203–7, doi: 10.1093/bja/77.2.203.

Mandal, S., V. K. Sinha, and N. Goyal. "Efficacy of Ketamine Therapy in the Treatment of Depression." *Indian Journal of Psychiatry* 61, no. 5 (2019): 480, doi: 10.4103/psychiatry.IndianJPsychiatry_484_18.

Martin, L. L., R. L. Bouchal, and D. J. Smith. "Ketamine Inhibits Serotonin Uptake in Vivo." *Neuropharmacology* 21, no. 2 (1982): 113–18, doi: 10.1016/0028-3908(82)90149-6.

Martinotti, G., et al. "Therapeutic Potentials of Ketamine and Esketamine in Obsessive-Compulsive Disorder (OCD), Substance Use Disorders (SUD) and Eating Disorders (ED): A Review of the Current Literature." *Brain Sciences* 11, no. 7 (2021): 856, doi: 10.3390/brainsci11070856.

Mason, N. L., et al. "Me, Myself, Bye: Regional Alterations in Glutamate and the Experience of Ego Dissolution with Psilocybin." *Neuropsychopharmacology* 45, no. 12 (2020): 2003–11, doi: 10.1038/s41386-020-0718-8.

McElvery, Raleigh. "The Past, Present and Future of Using Ketamine to Treat Depression." *Smithsonian Magazine*. May 24, 2022. www.smithsonianmag .com/science-nature/a-brief-history-of-ketamines-use-to-treat -depression-180980106.

McKoy, Jillian. "Depression Rates in US Tripled When the Pandemic First Hit —Now, They're Even Worse." Boston University. October 7, 2021. www .bu.edu/articles/2021/depression-rates-tripled-when-pandemic-first-hit.

McIntyre, Roger S., et al. "Synthesizing the Evidence for Ketamine and Esketamine in Treatment-Resistant Depression: An International Expert Opinion on the Available Evidence and Implementation." *American Journal of Psychiatry* 178, no. 5 (Mar. 17, 2021). doi.org: 10.1176/appi.ajp .2020.20081251.

Meglio, Marco. "FDA Approves IND for Ketamine in Parkinson Disease Dyskinesia." *Neurology Live*. May 24, 2021. www.neurologylive.com/view /fda-approves-ind-ketamine-parkinson-disease-dyskinesia.

Microdose Psychedelic Insights. "PharmaTher Granted FDA Orphan Drug Status for Ketamine." *Microdose*. February 2, 2022. https://microdose .buzz/news/pharmather-granted-fda-orphan-drug-status-for-ketamine.

Microdose Psychedelic Insights. "PharmaTher Receives FDA Approval for Ketamine Phase 2 Trial." *Microdose*. January 13, 2022. microdose.buzz /news/pharmather-receives-fda-approval-for-ketamine-phase-2-trial.

Minkove, Judy F. "Esketamine: A New Approach for Patients with Treatment -Resistant Depression." John Hopkins Medicine. September 26, 2019. www .hopkinsmedicine.org/news/articles/esketamine-a-new-approach-for -patients-with-treatment-resistant-depression.

Mitchell, Adam, Director of Clinical Research at My Self Wellness. Interview with Author. November 18, 2022.

Moaddel, R., et al. "Sub-Anesthetic Concentrations of (R,S)-Ketamine Metabolites Inhibit Acetylcholine-Evoked Currents in α7 Nicotinic

Acetylcholine Receptors." *European Journal of Pharmacology* 698, no. 1–3 (2013): 228–34, doi: 10.1016/j.ejphar.2012.11.023.

Monaco, Kristen. "How Effective Is Intranasal Esketamine, Really?" Med Page Today. May 21, 2019. www.medpagetoday.com/meetingcoverage/apa /79951.

Moore, Karenza, and Fiona Measham. "It's the Most Fun You Can Have for Twenty Quid": Motivations, Consequences and Meanings of British Ketamine Use." *Addiction Research and Theory* 16, no. 3 (Feb. 1, 2008).

Najum, Jason. "Heading to Phase 3? PharmaTher Announces Positive Results for Ketamine Trial." *Microdose*. March 23, 2022. microdose.buzz/news /moving-to-phase-3-pharmather-announces-positive-results-for -ketamine-trial.

Najum, Jason. "PharmaTher Granted Patent for Ketamine and Parkinson's." *Microdose*. July 13, 2022. microdose.buzz/news/pharmather-granted -patent-for-ketamine-and-parkinson-s.

Nakao, Mutsuhiro et al. "Cognitive-Behavioral Therapy for Management of Mental Health and Stress-Related Disorders: Recent Advances in Techniques and Technologies." *BioPsychoSocial Medicine* 15, no. 1 (Oct. 3, 2021): 16, doi: 10.1186/s13030-021-00219-w.

Nandan, Neethu K. et al. ""Esketamine" in Borderline Personality Disorder: A Look Beyond Suicidality." *Cureus* 14, no. 4 (April 30, 2022): e24632. doi: 10.7759/cureus.24632.

Nazeer, Dr. Abid. November 25, 2022. MD, FASAM. Psychiatrist with double board certifications in both psychiatry and addiction medicine.

*New York Times*. "Skull of Marcia Moore, Seattle Psychic, Found." *New York Times*. March 26, 1983. www.nytimes.com/1981/03/26/obituaries/skull-of -marcia-moore-seattle-psychic-found.html.

Newscope Capital Corporation. "PharmaTher Advancing Research for Novel Microneedle Delivery of Ketamine." PR Newswire. March 24, 2021. www .prnewswire.com/news-releases/pharmather-advancing-research -for-novel-microneedle-delivery-of-ketamine-301254671.html?utm_ source=pocket_reader.

Nour, Matthew M. et al. "Ego-Dissolution and Psychedelics: Validation of the Ego-Dissolution Inventory (EDI)." *Frontiers in Human Neuroscience* 10 (June 14, 2016): 269, doi:10.3389/fnhum.2016.00269.

NPR Staff. "The '60s Are Gone, But Psychedelic Research Trip Continues." *NPR*. March 9, 2014. https://www.npr.org/2014/03/09/288285764/the-60s -are-gone-but-psychedelic-research-trip-continues.

THE KETAMINE HANDBOOK

Oberhaus, Daniel. "This Nasal Spray Will Totally Change the Antidepressant Market." *VICE.* September 19, 2017. www.vice.com/en/article/wjxd9b /ketamine-nasal-spray-will-totally-change-the-market-for-antidepressant -drugs.

Ota, K. T., et al. "REDD1 Is Essential for Stress-Induced Synaptic Loss and Depressive Behavior." *Nature Medicine* 20, no. 5 (2014): 531–35, doi: 10.1038/nm.3513.

Pai, A., and M. Heining. "Ketamine." *Continuing Education in Anaesthesia Critical Care & Pain* 7, no. 2 (2007): 59–63, doi: 10.1093/bjaceaccp /mkm008.

Passie, Torsten, et al. "Comparative Effects of (S)-Ketamine and Racemic (R/S)-Ketamine on Psychopathology, State of Consciousness and Neurocognitive Performance in Healthy Volunteers." *European Neuropsychopharmacology* 44 (March 2, 2021): 92–104. www .sciencedirect.com/science/article/abs/pii/S0924977X21000079.

Pastrak, M., et al. "Systematic Review of the Use of Intravenous Ketamine for Fibromyalgia." *Ochsner Journal* 21, no. 4 (2021): 387–94, doi: 10.31486 /toj.21.0038.

Patti, Charles, Chief Brand Officer at My Self Wellness. Interview with Author. November 18, 2022.

Perry, E. B., et al. "Psychiatric Safety of Ketamine in Psychopharmacology Research." *Psychopharmacology* 192, no. 2 (2007): 253–60, doi: 10.1007 /s00213-007-0706-2.

Pomarol-Clotet, E. et al. "Psychological Effects of Ketamine in Healthy Volunteers. Phenomenological Study." *The British Journal of Psychiatry* 189 (2006): 173–97, doi: 10.1192/bjp.bp.105.015263.

Popoli, M., Z. Yan, B. S. EcEwen, and G. Sanacora. "The Stressed Synapse: The Impact of Stress and Glucocorticoids on Glutamate Transmission." *Nature Reviews Neuroscience* 13, no. 1 (2011): 22–37, doi: 10.1038/nrn3138.

Press Association. "Ketamine Made Illegal after Health Concerns." *The Guardian.* December 28, 2005. www.theguardian.com/society/2005/dec /29/drugsandalcohol.drugs.

Price, Rebecca B., et al. "A Novel, Brief, Fully Automated Intervention to Extend the Antidepressant Effect of a Single Ketamine Infusion: A Randomized Clinical Trial." *American Journal of Psychiatry* 178, no. 5 (September 2022): 383–99, doi.org:10.1176/appi.ajp.20220216.

Price, R. B., M. K. Nock, D. S. Charney, and S. J. Mathew. "Effects of Intravenous Ketamine on Explicit and Implicit Measures of Suicidality in

Treatment-Resistant Depression." *Biological Psychiatry* 66, no. 5 (2009): 522–26, doi: 10.1016/j.biopsych.2009.04.029.

Ragnhildstveit, A., et al. "Ketamine as a Novel Psychopharmacotherapy for Eating Disorders: Evidence and Future Directions." *Brain Sciences* 12, no. 3 (2022): 382, doi: 10.3390/brainsci12030382.

Ramanujan, Krishna. "Study Finds Tiny Brain Area Controls Work for Rewards." *Cornell Chronicle*. August 31, 2022. news.cornell.edu/stories /2022/08/study-finds-tiny-brain-area-controls-work-rewards.

Ramos, Marco A., et al. "Opinion: The New Ketamine-Based Antidepressant Is a Rip-Off." *VICE*. May 17, 2019. www.vice.com/en/article/pajkjy/opinion -the-new-ketamine-based-antidepressant-is-a-rip-off.

Rashmi, D., R. Zanan, S. John, K. Khandagale, and A. Nadaf. "Chapter 13–γ-Aminobutyric Acid (GABA): Biosynthesis, Role, Commercial Production, and Applications." *ScienceDirect* 57 (2018): 413–52. www .sciencedirect.com/science/article/abs/pii/B9780444640574000132 ?via%3Dihub.

Reddit user u/EER_ESQ. "My Ketamine Infusion Journey." February 2019. https://www.reddit.com/r/TherapeuticKetamine/comments/b3xcqf /my_ketamine_infusion_journey.

Reddit user u/manwithninebuttocks. "First Ketamine Infusion: Before and After." February 2019. https://www.reddit.com/r/TherapeuticKetamine /comments/bs8dv0/first_ketamine_infusion_before_and_after.

Reddit user u/madscribbler. "Long term success report (part 2)." January 1, 2022. https://www.reddit.com/r/TherapeuticKetamine/comments /pg247c/long_term_success_report_part_2.

Reddit user u/ocean6csgo. "My Ketamine Therapy Experience (Full Write-Up, Newbie Friendly)." October 1, 2022. https://www.reddit.com /r/TherapeuticKetamine/comments/y9hm3h/my_ketamine_therapy _experience_full_writeup.

Reddit user u/0ldboy67. "First infusion today, detailed description. AMA." February 6, 2018. https://www.reddit.com/r/TherapeuticKetamine /comments/936c60/first_infusion_today_detailed_description_ama.

Reynolds, Lauren Mackenzie. "A Brief History of Psychedelic Research." *Massive Science*, July 24, 2018, massivesci.com/articles/drug-excerpt -psychedelics-research-ban.

Robison, Dr. Reid, Chief Medical Officer for Numinus. Interview with Author. December 6, 2022. MD MBA. Chief Medical Officer for Numinus.

Robson, Steve. "Superhuman Man "High on PCP" Beats Woman Cop Unconscious and Fights off TEN More." *Mirror UK*. October 15, 2016. www

.mirror.co.uk/news/world-news/man-high-pcp-shows-superhuman
-9049594.

Rodriguez, C. I., et al. "Randomized Controlled Crossover Trial of
Ketamine in Obsessive-Compulsive Disorder: Proof-of-Concept."
*Neuropsychopharmacology* 38, no. 12 (2013): 2475–83, doi: 10.1038
/npp.2013.150.

Romeo, B., et al. "Meta-Analysis of Short- and Mid-Term Efficacy of Ketamine
in Unipolar and Bipolar Depression." *Psychiatry Research* 230, no. 2 (2015):
682–88, doi: 10.1016/j.psychres.2015.10.032.

Rose, N. "Neuroscience and the Future for Mental Health?" *Epidemiology and
Psychiatric Sciences* 25, no. 2 (2015): 95–100, doi:  10.1017
/s2045796015000621.

Rothberg, R. L., et al. "Mystical-Type Experiences Occasioned by Ketamine
Mediate Its Impact on At-Risk Drinking: Results from a Randomized,
Controlled Trial." *Journal of Psychopharmacology* 35, no. 2 (2020): 150–58,
doi: 10.1177/0269881120970879.

Saligan, L. N., D. A. Luckenbaugh, E. E. Slonena, R. Machado-Vieira, and C. A.
Zarate, Jr. "An Assessment of the Anti-Fatigue Effects of Ketamine from a
Double-Blind, Placebo-Controlled, Crossover Study in Bipolar Disorder."
*Journal of Affective Disorders* 194 (2016): 115–19, doi: 10.1016/j.jad.2016
.01.009.

Sartim, A. G., K. M. Silveira, P. H. Gobira, F. S. Guimaraes, G. Wegener, and
S. R. Joca. "Co-Administration of Cannabidiol and Ketamine Induces
Antidepressant-Like Effects Devoid of Hyperlocomotor Side-Effects."
*Neuropharmacology* 195 (2021): 108679, doi: 10.1016/j.neuropharm.2021
.108679.

Schatzberg, A. F. "A Word to the Wise about Intranasal Esketamine." *American
Journal of Psychiatry* 176, no. 6 (2019): 422–24, doi: 10.1176/appi.ajp.2019
.19040423.

Scheidegger, M., et al. "Ketamine Decreases Resting State Functional Network
Connectivity in Healthy Subjects: Implications for Antidepressant Drug
Action." *PLOS One* 7, no. 9 (2012): e44799, doi: 10.1371/journal.pone
.0044799.

Schenberg, Eduardo Ekman. "Psychedelic-Assisted Psychotherapy: A
Paradigm Shift in Psychiatric Research and Development." *Frontiers in
Pharmacology* 9 (Jul. 5, 2018): 733, doi: 10.3389/fphar.2018.00733.

Serafini, G., R. H. Howland, F. Rovedi, P. Girardi, and M. Amore. "The Role
of Ketamine in Treatment-Resistant Depression: A Systematic Review."

*Current Neuropharmacology* 12, no. 5 (2014): 444–61, doi: 10.2174/157015
9x12666140619204251.

Shin, C., and Y. Kim. "Ketamine in Major Depressive Disorder: Mechanisms
and Future Perspectives." *Psychiatry Investigation* 17, no. 3 (2020): 181–92,
doi: 10.30773/pi.2019.0236.

Short, B., J. Fong, V. Galvez, W. Shelker, and C. K. Loo. "Side-Effects Associated
with Ketamine Use in Depression: A Systematic Review." *Lancet Psychiatry*
5, no. 1 (2018): 65–78, doi: 10.1016/s2215-0366(17)30272-9.

Silverman, Ed. "J&J's New Esketamine Drug for Depression May Solve an
Unmet Need, but May Not Be Cost-Effective." STAT News. March 22,
2019. www.statnews.com/pharmalot/2019/03/22/antidepressants-cost
-effective-johnson-and-johnson.

Singh, J. B., et al. "A Double-Blind, Randomized, Placebo-Controlled,
Dose-Frequency Study of Intravenous Ketamine in Patients with
Treatment-Resistant Depression." *American Journal of Psychiatry* 173, no.
8 (2016): 816–26, doi: 10.1176/appi.ajp.2016.16010037.

Singh, Jaskaran, and Ivo Caers. "Esketamine for the Treatment of Treatment
-Refractory or Treatment-Resistant Depression." *Google Patents.* patents
.google.com/patent/US20130236573A1/en.

Sleigh, J., M. Harvey, L. Voss, and B. Denny. "Ketamine—More Mechanisms of
Action than Just NMDA Blockade." *Trends in Anaesthesia and Critical Care*
4, no. 2-3 (2014): 76–81, doi: 10.1016/j.tacc.2014.03.002.

Sofia, R. D., and J. J. Harakal. "Evaluation of Ketamine HCl for Anti
-Depressant Activity." *Archives Internationales de Pharmacodynamie et de
Therapie* 214, no. 1 (1975): 68–74. pubmed.ncbi.nlm.nih.gov/1156026.

Stanford, John A., et al. "Ketamine Prolongs Survival in Symptomatic
SOD1-G93A Mice." *RRNMF Neuromuscular Journal* 2, no. 2 (May 27, 2021):
doi: 10.17161/rrnmf.v2i2.15108.

Stone, D. M., et al. "Vital Signs: Trends in State Suicide Rates–United States,
1999–2016 and Circumstances Contributing to Suicide–27 States, 2015."
*Morbidity and Mortality Weekly Report* 67, no. 22 (2018): 617–24, doi:
10.15585/mmwr.mm6722a1.

Stone, M. B., Z. S. Yaseen, B. J. Miller, K. Richardville, S. N. Kalaria, and I.
Kirsch. "Response to Acute Monotherapy for Major Depressive Disorder
in Randomized, Placebo Controlled Trials Submitted to the US Food and
Drug Administration: Individual Participant Data Analysis." *BMJ* (2022):
e067606, doi: 10.1136/bmj-2021-067606.

Strassman R. J., C. R. Qualls. "Dose-Response Study of N,N-
Dimethyltryptamine in Humans: I. Neuroendocrine, Autonomic, and

Cardiovascular Effects." *Arch Gen Psychiatry* 51, no. 2 (1994):85–97, doi: 10.1001/archpsyc.1994.03950020009001.

Strous, J. F. M., et al. "Brain Changes Associated with Long-Term Ketamine Abuse, a Systematic Review." *Frontiers in Neuroanatomy* 16 (2022), doi: 10.3389/fnana.2022.795231.

Thielking, Megan. "The Psychiatry Field Is Buzzing with Anticipation—and Hesitation—about Esketamine for Depression." STAT News. February 20, 2019. www.statnews.com/2019/02/20/psychiatry-awaits-esketamine -with-excitement-hesitation.

Thompson, S. L., et al. "Ketamine Induces Immediate and Delayed Alterations of OCD-like Behavior." *Psychopharmacology* 237, no. 3 (2020) 627–38, doi: 10.1007/s00213-019-05397-8.

Traber, D. L., R. Wilson, and L. Priano. "Differentiation of the Cardiovascular Effects of CI-581." *Anesthesia & Analgesia* 47, no. 6 (1968): 769. journals .lww.com/anesthesia-analgesia/Citation/1968/11000/Differentiation_of _the_Cardiovascular_Effects_of.25.aspx.

US Department of Justice. "Drug-Facilitated Sexual Assault DEA Victim Witness Assistance Program." https://www.dea.gov/sites/default /files/2018-07/DFSA_0.PDF.

US Food and Drug Administration. "FDA Approves New Nasal Spray Medication for Treatment-Resistant Depression; Available Only at a Certified Doctor's Office or Clinic." FDA. March 24, 2020. www.fda.gov /news-events/press-announcements/fda-approves-new-nasal-spray -medication-treatment-resistant-depression-available-only -certified#:~:text=The%20efficacy%20of%20Spravato%20was.

van der Schier, R., M. Roozekrans, M. van Velzen, A. Dahan, and M. Niesters. "Opioid-Induced Respiratory Depression: Reversal by Non-opioid Drugs." *F1000Prime Reports* 6, no. 79 (2014), doi: 10.12703/p6-79.

van Gerven, J., and A. Cohen. "Vanishing Clinical Psychopharmacology." *British Journal of Clinical Pharmacology* 72, no. 1 (2011): 1–5, doi: 10.1111/j.1365-2125.2011.04021.x.

Vincent, Isabel. "Was Vanished Heiress Marcia Moore Murdered—or 'Dematerialized'?" *New York Post*. December 18, 2021. nypost.com/2021 /12/18/was-vanished-heiress-marcia-moore-murdered-or-dematerialized.

Vollenweider, F. "Positron Emission Tomography and Fluorodeoxyglucose Studies of Metabolic Hyperfrontality and Psychopathology in the Psilocybin Model of Psychosis." *Neuropsychopharmacology* 16, no. 5 (1997): 357–72, doi: 10.1016/s0893-133x(96)00246-1.

Vollenweider, F. X., and M. Kometer. "The Neurobiology of Psychedelic Drugs: Implications for the Treatment of Mood Disorders." *Nature Reviews Neuroscience* 11, no. 9 (2010): 642–51, doi: 10.1038/nrn2884.

Wang, P., et al. "Mediating Role of Rumination and Negative Affect in the Effect of Mind-Wandering on Symptoms in Patients with Obsessive-Compulsive Disorder." *Frontiers in Psychiatry* 12 (2021): 755159, doi: 10.3389/fpsyt.2021.755159.

Weil, Andrew T. "The Strange Case of the Harvard Drug Scandal." *Look Magazine*. November 5, 1963. Psychedelic Library. www.psychedelic-library.org/look1963.htm.

Weisman, H. "Anesthesia for Pediatric Ophthalmology." *Annals of Ophthalmology* 3 (1971): 229–32. PMID: 5163952.

White, P. F., J. Schuttler, A. Shafer, D.R. Stanski, Y. Horai, and A. J. Trevor. "Comparative Pharmacology of the Ketamine Isomers." *British Journal of Anaesthesia* 57, no. 2 (1985): 197–203, doi: 10.1093/bja/57.2.197.

Wilkinson, S. T., et al. "The Effect of a Single Dose of Intravenous Ketamine on Suicidal Ideation: A Systematic Review and Individual Participant Data Meta-Analysis." *The American Journal of Psychiatry* 175, no. 2 (2018): 150–58, doi: 10.1176/appi.ajp.2017.17040472.

Williams, N. R., et al. "Attenuation of Antidepressant Effects of Ketamine by Opioid Receptor Antagonism." *American Journal of Psychiatry* 175, no. 12 (2018): 1205–15, doi: 10.1176/appi.ajp.2018.18020138.

Wink, L. K., et al. "Brief Report: Intranasal Ketamine in Adolescents and Young Adults with Autism Spectrum Disorder–Initial Results of a Randomized, Controlled, Crossover, Pilot Study." *Journal of Autism and Developmental Disorders* 51, no. 4 (2020): 1392–99, doi: 10.1007/s10803-020-04542-z.

Witt, Emily. "Ketamine Therapy Is Going Mainstream. Are We Ready?" *The New Yorker*. December 29, 2021. https://www.newyorker.com/culture/annals-of-inquiry/ketamine-therapy-is-going-mainstream-are-we-ready.

Xiong, Z., et al. "Neuronal Brain Injury after Cerebral Ischemic Stroke Is Ameliorated after Subsequent Administration of (R)-Ketamine, but Not (S)-Ketamine." *Pharmacology, Biochemistry, and Behavior* 191 (2020): 172904, doi: 10.1016/j.pbb.2020.172904.

Yale University. "A Randomized Active Placebo Controlled Trial of Ketamine in Borderline Personality Disorder." ClinicTrials.gov. Last updated June 1, 2022. clinicaltrials.gov/ct2/show/NCT03395314.

Yanagihara, Y., et al. "Plasma Concentration Profiles of Ketamine and Norketamine after Administration of Various Ketamine Preparations to

Healthy Japanese Volunteers." *Biopharmaceutics & Drug Disposition* 24, no. 1 (2002): 37–43, doi: 10.1002/bdd.336.

Yang, Yan, et al. "Ketamine Blocks Bursting in the Lateral Habenula to Rapidly Relieve Depression." *Nature* 554, no. 7692 (2018): 317–22, doi: 10.1038 /nature25509.

Zand, Dr. Sam. BetterUCare.com. https://www.betterucare.com/resources /meet-the-team.

Zanos, Panos, et al. "Ketamine and Ketamine Metabolite Pharmacology: Insights into Therapeutic Mechanisms." *Pharmacological Reviews* 70, no. 3 (2018): 621–60, doi: 10.1124/pr.117.015198.

Zarate, Carlos A., et al. "Relationship of Ketamine's Plasma Metabolites with Response, Diagnosis, and Side Effects in Major Depression." *Biological Psychiatry* 72, no. 4 (2012): 331–38, doi: 10.1016/j.biopsych.2012.03.004.

Zhang, Ji-chun, Su-xia Li, and Kenji Hashimoto. "R (−)-Ketamine Shows Greater Potency and Longer Lasting Antidepressant Effects than S (+)-Ketamine." *Pharmacology Biochemistry and Behavior* 116 (2014): 137–41, doi: 10.1016/j.pbb.2013.11.033.

Zhdanava, Maryia, et al. "The Prevalence and National Burden of Treatment -Resistant Depression and Major Depressive Disorder in the United States." *The Journal of Clinical Psychiatry* 82, no. 2 (2021), doi: 10.4088 /jcp.20m13699.

Zimmerman, Andrew W. "Treating Autism and Other Developmental Disorders in Children with NMDA Receptor Antagonists." *Google Patents*. patents.google.com/patent/US4994467A/en.

# INDEX

sildenafil citrate (Viagra), 49
Smith Ketamine Services, 101
Special K. *See* ketamine
Spravato, 18–22, 47
  controversy, 18–21
  efficacy of, 25
  esketamine, 63, 65, 79, 102, 104
  ethical concerns, 21–22
  intranasal administration, 50–51
  Johnson & Johnson, 106
Spravato provider finder tool, 96
Stevens, Calvin, 8
stopping-off effect, 23
sympathetic nervous system, 32–34
sympathomimetic agent, 52
synaptogenesis, 40
systemic effect, 52–54
  cardiovascular, 52–53
  neurological, 54
  pulmonary, 53–54

# T

telehealth esketamine, 79–80
telehealth services, ethical concerns
of, 109–110
therapeutic applications, 56–71
  analgesic agent, 63
  anesthetic agent, 62
    dosing, 62–63
  anti-inflammatory effects, 68–69
  antidepressant, 64–65
  antidepressants, 57–59
  depression and dosing, 68
  microdosing, 64
  psychiatry, crisis in, 60–61
therapeutic ketamine, 100
traditional psychedelics, 10
tranquilizer, defined, 29
transcranial magnetic stimulation
(TMS), 98

Trip Sitter Options, 109
TripSitter.Clinic, 106–107

# U

US Department of Justice, 114

# W

Wondermed, 108
work with your insurance, 97–99
World Health Organization, 56

# Z

ZAND, SAM, 74, 78, 83, 93, 94, 102,
122

# ACKNOWLEDGMENTS

Thank you to Ulysses Press for this life-changing opportunity and for all of the wonderful work you put out into the world.

Thanks to the team of talented doctors I interviewed who graciously donated their time and valuable insights to help, and the publicists who very kindly connected me to them.

To my mom: thanks for everything, for passing on your strength, determination, and ambition. I admire you so much.

To Nemo: thanks for being there for me and encouraging me at every step.

To all the artists whose works inspired me to keep going when I was at my lowest: thank you for lifting me up.

To the kind, diligent health-care providers who fought for me in Oregon: thank you from the bottom of my heart. Words cannot express how grateful I am for your care.

Thanks to Dr. Constance Ohlinger and Dr. Eli Thompson, who saved my life in more ways than I can count.

Thanks to the most incredible therapist a girl could ask for, Linda Farhat, who helped my broken heart grieve and heal.

And thank you to every doctor, researcher, scientist, therapist, nurse practitioner, medical professional, educator, and healer who helped make this work possible. I love you all, and wish you nothing but the best. Blessed be.

# THE KETAMINE HANDBOOK

A Beginner's Guide to Ketamine–
Assisted Therapy for Depression,
Anxiety, Trauma, PTSD, and More

# JANELLE
# LASSALLE

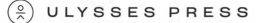 ULYSSES PRESS

Published by:
Uysses Press
PO Box 3440
Berkeley, CA 94703
www.ulyssespress.com

ISBN: 978-1-64604-502-0
Library of Congress Control Number: 2023930761

Printed in the United States by Versa Press
10  9  8  7  6  5  4  3  2  1

Acquisitions editor: Casie Vogel
Managing editor: Claire Chun
Project editor: Renee Rutledge
Proofreader: Beret Olsen
Front cover design: Elke Barter
Interior design and layout: Winnie Liu
Indexer: S4Carlisle
Author photo: © Nehemiah Chen

# ABOUT THE AUTHOR

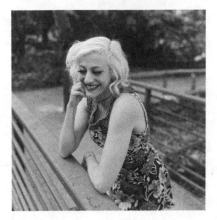

Janelle Lassalle is a freelance writer and artist who specializes in producing cannabis and psychedelic content. Much of her work is data driven and research oriented, highlighting the therapeutic promise and potential of cannabinoids and other psychedelics as they continue to emerge. Janelle has produced psychedelic content for a number of leading industry names including Field Trip, Psychedelic Support, and Mind Cure. You can find her writing in a number of top-tier publications, including *Forbes* and *Rolling Stone*, by taking a peek at her website LassalleWorks.com or checking out her psychedelic-inspired artwork over at her Instagram @jenkhari.